"Will is Dr. Fiber! Get on the fiber train and transform your health from the inside out, literally. . . . Poop like a champ, build an immune system that is a fortress, and feed your brain premium-grade fuel. Pick up a copy of *Fiber Fueled* today!"

—**Rip Esselstyn,** *New York Times* **bestselling author of** *The Engine 2 Diet*

"This book is a timely and authoritative discussion of the overwhelming scientific evidence supporting the health benefits of a largely plant based diet. It focuses on the role of fiber, a key element of plant-based diets, and presents this ancient wisdom from the perspective of modern microbiome science. A must-read for everybody still unconvinced about the best diet to stay healthy."

—**Emeran A. Mayer, MD, PhD, author of** *The Mind-Gut Connection* **and Distinguished Professor of Medicine, Physiology and Psychiatry, David Geffen School of Medicine at UCLA**

"The gut microbiome is the engine that drives the body to health and today's diet is deficient in its preferred fuel: fiber, the elixir of life. Instead, we are overfed, undernourished, and overmedicated. *Fiber Fueled* is a must-have owner's manual revealing the secrets for gut and total body health. Read Dr. Will Bulsiewicz's groundbreaking book today!"

—**Gerard E. Mullin, MD, MS, author of** *The Gut Balance Revolution* **and Director of Integrative GI Nutrition Services, Johns Hopkins Medicine**

"Like the microbes in our gut, Dr. Bulsiewicz helps us digest a large quantity of complex material. *Fiber Fueled* translates the latest cutting-edge science of the gut microbiome into accessible and practical information. This is required reading whether you are interested in a heathier gut and body or learning about one of the most transformational fields in biomedicine."

—**Justin Sonnenburg, PhD, author of** *The Good Gut* **and Associate Professor, Stanford University**

"If 'all disease begins in the gut' as Hippocrates said, then all health begins there too. Dr. Bulsiewicz and the Fiber Fueled 4 Week Plan are the natural jumpstart to feeding our gut its preferred and premium fuel. This book is the answer for so many of my patients searching for a higher level of wellness."

—**Joel Kahn, MD, FACC, author of** *The Plant-Based Solution* **and Clinical Professor, Wayne State University School of Medicine**

"Drawing on his vast experience as a practicing gastroenterologist, Dr. Bulsiewicz illuminates a path to optimal gut health using 'food as medicine' to unleash the incredibly powerful, absolutely fascinating, and wildly underrated postbiotics called short-chain fatty acids. It's worked for him, it's worked for his patients, and it can work for you too."

—**Mahmoud A. Ghannoum, PhD, MBA, author of** *Total Gut Balance* **and Director of the Center for Medical Mycology, Case Western Reserve University**

"Although I've actively investigated intestinal bacterial functions my entire career, I found Dr. B's *Fiber Fueled* book both highly informative and inspiring. It brings fresh perspectives and very practical solutions to vexing clinical problems that can be reversed and prevented by incorporating the lifelong healthy eating patterns described in this transformative book."

—**R. Balfour Sartor, MD, Co-Director, Center for Gastrointestinal Biology and Disease, Midget Distinguished Professor of Medicine, Microbiology & Immunology, University of North Carolina School of Medicine**

"*Fiber Fueled* is what happens when you combine almost two decades of medical training, an unrivaled passion for helping people live healthier, and an incredible ability to break down complex science into easy-to-digest information for everyone to access. Far more than a diet book—a true master class in gut health that will be hard to put down."

—**Simon Hill, master's of nutrition, host of the** *Plant Proof Podcast,* **and author of** *The Proof Is in the Plants*

"At a time when many 'experts' are peddling the latest fad diets, Americans are justifiably confused about what to eat. Will has used his considerable skills to provide an engaging, evidence-based guide that makes it clear that when you optimize your gut microbiota through diet and lifestyle, you also improve your health."

—**Nicholas J. Shaheen, MD, MPH, Chief of Gastroenterology & Hepatology, Bozymski-Heizer Distinguished Professor of Medicine, University of North Carolina School of Medicine**

"Gastroenterologists should focus on diet and lifestyle to prevent and reverse disease and only use pills and procedures when these less invasive interventions fail. Dr. Bulsiewicz provides an excellent blueprint in his book, *Fiber Fueled*, for a more patient-centered approach to improve overall health."

—**John Pandolfino, MD, MSCI, Chief of Gastroenterology & Hepatology, Hans Popper Professor of Medicine, Northwestern University**

"After many decades of physiological studies evaluating how the GI system works in health and disease, it is only in the last decade that food, fiber, diet, and the microbiome has found its proper scientific place. Using his extensive experience, Dr. Bulsiewicz has compiled this new knowledge into a clear and concise book so that readers having GI illness or who are in health can truly benefit."

—**Douglas A. Drossman, MD, Drossman Gastroenterology, President Emeritus and COO of the Rome Foundation, and Professor Emeritus of Medicine and Psychiatry, University of North Carolina School of Medicine**

"We live in a country where most people eat twice the recommended daily allowance of protein and almost no one is eating the recommended fiber. Many think that because we do not absorb fiber it cannot be important. Dr. Bulsiewicz combines his firsthand knowledge with the available science to teach the reader the importance of eating varied forms of fiber to feed our varied forms of bacteria residing in our gut, and in turn improve and prevent both systemic diseases and gut pathology. And if you think your gut just can't tolerate fiber, do not fear. The good doctor has a whole chapter dedicated to helping you get over bloating and other symptoms commonly associated with high-fiber diets."

—**Garth Davis MD, author of *Proteinaholic* and bariatric surgeon & Medical Director of Weight Management, Mission Hospital, Asheville, North Carolina**

"In a world where most people are obsessed about consuming a lot of protein, this book will revolutionize the way you think about nutrition. In this evidence-based book, Dr. B delineates the importance of fiber for great gut health. I recommend for everyone to read this book as great health begins in your gut."

—**Angie Sadeghi, MD, author of *The Trifecta of Health***

FIBER
FUELED

*The Plant-Based Gut Health Program
for Losing Weight, Restoring Your Health,
and Optimizing Your Microbiome*

WILL BULSIEWICZ, MD, MSCI

AVERY
an imprint of Penguin Random House
New York

AVERY

an imprint of Penguin Random House LLC
penguinrandomhouse.com

Most Avery books are available at special quantity discounts for bulk purchase
for sales promotions, premiums, fund-raising, and educational needs. Special
books or book excerpts also can be created to fit specific needs. For details,
write SpecialMarkets@penguinrandomhouse.com.

ISBN 9780593084564
eBook ISBN 9780593084571

Printed in the United States of America
16th Printing

Book design by Renato Stanisic

The recipes contained in this book are to be followed exactly as written. The
publisher is not responsible for your specific health or allergy needs that may
require medical supervision. The publisher is not responsible for any adverse
reactions to the recipes contained in this book.

Neither the publisher nor the author is engaged in rendering professional advice
or services to the individual reader. The ideas, procedures, and suggestions
contained in this book are not intended as a substitute for consulting with your
physician. All matters regarding your health require medical supervision.
Neither the author nor the publisher shall be liable or responsible for any loss or
damage allegedly arising from any information or suggestion in this book.

I lost my dad during the preparation of this book.
It was sudden and completely unexpected.

I couldn't wait to share this book with him.
It would have been easy to just send an electronic copy,
but I really wanted his first read to be a physical book,
with the hardcover, all the pages,
and his son's name on the front.

Over the past few months, my dad repeatedly told me
how proud he was of me. He told me that my grandparents John
and Helen Bulsiewicz would have been so proud of the work
I was doing in the name of our family. I can't tell you how
much it means to me that he said all that.

It breaks my heart that he's not here anymore.
I am who I am because of him. But I will forever
be grateful for the special times that we shared.

Love you, Dad. Will always be thinking of you.
This book is for you.

Contents

Author's Note

*D*ear Friends,

My goal with this book is to send you off on a journey that transforms your life. I want you healthier and happier, and I truly believe that the words on these pages will guide you to that better place.

There was only one way to accomplish my goal, and that was to make this book a celebration of scientific discovery. We want the laws of nature working for us, not against us. Science becomes the compass that guides us to that better place. I share this because you will read this book and hopefully find it lighthearted and entertaining, but just know that if you pulled back the curtain you'd discover more than six hundred studies backing up those words. Legitimate, valid science is the reason accomplished scientists and doctors are unified in support of this book. You can review all of my references plus more details about my evidence-based approach at www.theplantfedgut.com /research.

With that said, being *Fiber Fueled* isn't a quick fix or a diet; it's a lifestyle trajectory that heals. In some cases, those lifestyle choices are optimal when personalized to your needs and bio-individuality. Therefore, the implementation of the practices in this book should be done under the guidance of a qualified health professional to ensure that your specific needs are being met.

Additionally, some of you may want to continue the conversation with me after reading this book or seek additional resources, and I welcome and celebrate that. Please join me at www.theplantfedgut .com, where you will find my podcasts, blog posts, social media channels, free email subscription, and online course that will allow you to go beyond the book.

Onward to health and happiness together!

Introduction

Leslie came into my office worn out and exasperated. She was thirty-six years old, but she felt like she was pushing eighty. She was overweight, a trend that started in her late twenties while taking the antibiotic minocycline for her acne. She struggled daily with fatigue, sluggishness, insomnia, and lack of motivation. Her skin was broken out, her hair was thinning, and she had persistent loose stools. On top of all this was her extensive list of medical ailments: irritable bowel, type 2 diabetes, hyperlipidemia, autoimmune thyroiditis, depression, and anxiety.

After seeing several other GI doctors, a chiropractor, a hormone specialist, and an expensive cash-only functional doctor, she was confused and frustrated by the conflicting recommendations. Here she was at thirty-six, on four different medications with ten supplements to boot. "This isn't the life I envisioned for myself," she told me on that first visit. "I'm way too young to be feeling this old."

Much of her frustration stemmed from not knowing what to eat. What should have been simple had become so complicated. She had gone Paleo in her late twenties to combat weight gain and she soon progressed to the Whole 30. She felt better for a short time on those diets, but when the weight gain and fatigue slowly started to creep back in, she desperately searched for a new diet solution and tried eliminating phytates and lectins. She'd been gluten-free for almost ten years and by the time I saw her in my office, she had completely eliminated grains, legumes, dairy, and nightshades. Her diet now consisted mostly of arugula, avocado, grass-fed meat, and bone broth, with very little variation. At times she'd test herself with some beans or whole-wheat bread, but she'd experience gas and bloating, which the diet gurus she was following warned was proof of inflammation.

"It is maddening to follow all the experts' recommendations religiously and do exactly as I'm told, only to feel worse than ever and see my weight fluctuate like a yo-yo!" she exclaimed. With each progressive elimination, she'd see at most short-term improvement, only to slide back into the same exhaustive pattern. The last straw came when she tried the ketogenic diet to lose weight, but it just made her diarrhea worse and it was now a bigger problem than ever.

At this point in our conversation, she was physically slumped forward, elbows on her knees, staring at the ground, eyes welled up with tears. I pulled my chair closer to hers and leaned in so we were on the same eye level.

"Leslie, it's going to be all right. We're going to get you better." She looked up, a glimmer of hope in her eye. "I totally get your frustration. This is the most confusing time in human history for people who just want to get better. Too many experts saying too many different things. I need you to trust me. If you're with me, then this is rock bottom right here, right now. Today is a fresh start for you with a new approach that makes you feel better and restores the real version of yourself that has been missing these last few years."

Over the following months, Leslie and I worked closely together to make some major changes. We took her off most of her supplements and slowly reintroduced diversity back into her diet. Foods that she had been told were off-limits were brought back at the right time, in the right amount. She began to really enjoy her food for the first time in years. The restrictive diet had been challenging, boring, and futile for her. She got rid of her bone broth and tapered down on her animal product consumption while increasing fruits, veggies, and even whole grains. Artificial sweeteners and processed foods stayed on the sideline. Beans came back on the menu! And while the process wasn't always easy, we worked through it together.

Front and center in her new way of eating was fiber-rich plants—fruit, veggies, whole grains, beans, and legumes. Why fiber? Because as you're about to learn in this book, fiber is the heart and soul of true gut healing, and true gut healing leads to better health in everything from your cardiovascular system to your brain health to your hormonal health. It's really that powerful.

When Leslie emerged on the other side and settled into her new approach, she was beaming with energy. She was having fun experimenting with all the new foods that she'd previously eliminated. She now knew exactly which foods she was sensitive to and was able to include them in her diet on a regular basis by simply being careful with portion size. Twelve pounds had melted away. Meanwhile, getting *Fiber Fueled* reversed Leslie's diabetes and dramatically dropped her cholesterol. She was able to reduce the dosage of her thyroid medication, and she was back to having normal bowel movements. Best of all, she felt like herself again: alive, optimistic, and excited for the possibilities ahead of her.

Getting *Fiber Fueled* can help you with whatever you're struggling with, too, whether it's weight gain, hormone imbalances, digestive issues, or you just want to feel better in your own skin. I know this because I've seen it in Leslie and in hundreds of my own patients. Now it's your turn.

The *Fiber Fueled* program

Perhaps you're one of the many Americans suffering with digestive issues: heartburn, abdominal pain, gas and bloating, diarrhea or constipation. I know there are at least seventy million of you out there because I personally published that statistic in *Gastroenterology*, the top American journal in my field, just a few years ago. Without question, gut health starts with the foods that you eat. Unfortunately much of the advice being offered by popular "experts" is dead wrong. I've grown tired of watching bone broth and grass-fed meat be touted as gut healing. There's not a single study to support that, not even a crappy one. Instead of offering recommendations based on trends and pseudoscience, my program offers you a scientifically validated approach that will truly heal your gut by restoring order to your gut microbiome.

Do you have a sensitive stomach? Do you have trouble processing certain foods, like beans, broccoli, and gluten-containing grains? Food sensitivity has become a major issue worldwide, with an estimated 20 percent of the world's population suffering from some form of food intolerance. I see it every single day in my clinic, and I'm going to share with you the strategy I've devised for my own patients to help identify exactly which foods they are sensitive to. I'll also share my easy, step-by-step plan for how to reintroduce those foods to eliminate the sensitivity and get back to enjoying them again.

If you're one of the millions of Americans who have an autoimmune disease, then this book is for you, too. Seventy percent of the immune system resides in the gut, literally just a single layer of cells separating it from the microbiota. It's hard to separate the two—they rise and fall together. By optimizing your gut microbes, we can help get your immune system back on track.

Do you or someone you love have heart disease, cancer, a history of stroke, or Alzheimer's disease? These are just a few of the dangerous and all-too-common conditions that can improve with this plan. The

Fiber Fueled approach doesn't just benefit digestive disorders. In fact, this is literally the only diet plan that's been scientifically proven to actually reverse heart disease.

Maybe you consider yourself pretty healthy and just want to stay that way. That's the situation I'm in as well. I haven't always been in great shape, but right now, by practicing what I preach, I feel fantastic. I've lost nearly fifty pounds, I'm back to my college weight, and I feel like I've actually reversed the aging process. There's real science to support that. This is the only dietary approach shown to lengthen telomeres, which is the part of our cells that cause aging as they get shorter. Longer telomeres have been suggested to indicate slow aging and reduced risk of heart disease, cancer, Alzheimer's, and Parkinson's.

You're going to learn in this book that you are one of a kind with a gut microbiome as unique as a fingerprint. So there is no one-size-fits-all when it comes to diet. Something that works for another person may not work for you, and that's driven by the individual nature of your gut microbiome. But if you'll treat me like your doctor, mentor, and lifestyle coach, I'll walk you through a program that will be personalized and tailored to your unique needs and ultimately guide you to the vibrant health that you deserve.

This book is the consummation of everything I've learned about gut health during the two decades that I've been grinding to become the best doctor I can possibly be. With the Fiber Fueled 4 Weeks (see Chapter 10), I'll show you how to use a healthy diet, lifestyle, and high-quality supplements to address the root cause of your problems. This isn't just a treatment plan; it's a way of life that will help you discover your healthiest self. Your symptoms will dissipate, your doctor will be shocked when your medicine ends up in the trash, and you'll enjoy the vibrant health you've always wanted.

Sadly, I must admit that our health care system has failed you

When I was younger, it drove me nuts when people would say that health care in America sucks. I definitely took it personally. You have to understand, for sixteen years I toiled, sacrificed, and committed every last ounce of energy that I had to that "sucky" health care system. I took out huge loans so that I could go to Vanderbilt for undergrad and Georgetown for medical school. I worked six days a week, at work before sunrise and home after sunset, for what I calculated was less than minimum wage after medical school. My family would be off on vacation together, and I'd be on call in the hospital wearing the same boxer shorts I wore yesterday because I was too tired to do my laundry. (For the record, I don't do that anymore!)

But now I get it. There's a reason why the United States is ranked forty-third in the world in life expectancy. We have a health care system that's great at identifying problems once they exist and then trying to manage them with a combination of pills and procedures. Sure, we can improve symptoms or slow disease progression in some cases, but it always comes at a cost. It's sick care, not health care. There is little to no focus on prevention.

What we're missing is an acknowledgment that a couple of milligrams of medicine will *never* be able to overcome the effect of what we eat. Each of us consumes an average of three pounds of food per day. Keeping the math simple, that's one thousand pounds of food per year, meaning we'll each consume about eighty thousand pounds of food during our lifetimes. Somehow, our medical system doesn't want to acknowledge that these eighty thousand pounds of food matter, but I'm telling you right now: a few milligrams of medicine will never be more important than the eighty thousand pounds of food you eat. When we wait for disease to manifest, we've already missed our greatest opportunity. As Benjamin Franklin said, "An ounce of prevention is worth a pound of cure."

Simply put, the greatest determinant of your health during your lifetime is the food that you choose to eat. As it turns out, your diet is also the greatest determinant of the health of your microbiome. In other words, you could nourish your body with life-giving food and reap the rewards of better health. Or you can punish your body with poisons disguised as food that actually take health away with every bite.

Unfortunately, our health care system simply ignores the role of nutrition in health and disease. Consider medical education in the United States. Medical students spend months learning the nuances of drug pharmacology, but formal nutrition training can be just two weeks or less. For me, that training occurred during my second year of medical school. It would be more than ten years later that I would finally complete all of my training to be a licensed gastroenterologist. And during that entire ten years, it was never mentioned again.

And did you know that even if I provide nutritional counseling, there's no way for me as a gastroenterologist to bill for the time that I use to do that? Look, I'm not telling you this to say, "Pay me more!" I'm telling you this to say that our system actually penalizes doctors for taking the time to discuss nutrition. I'll use my office as an example. We currently have three doctors and about fifteen employees. That means that I am personally responsible for covering the salaries of five individuals before I see even a dime. So uncompensated time becomes rather costly. Sadly, this creates a major deterrent to most doctors incorporating nutrition into their practice.

For me, I've built a successful career by forgetting the money and the rules and just doing what's best for my patients. When I finished my training and went into practice for the first time, my patients would ask me fairly intuitive questions. "Dr. B., what should I eat so I don't get so much gas?" "Hey, Doc, what's the best food to prevent diarrhea?" "So I was wondering, can diet help me control my ulcerative colitis?" I have a strong, intrinsic motivation to provide the very best care for each person who walks through my office door, and I just couldn't stand having a patient ask me something like this and not be able to provide an answer.

While I was searching for answers to these questions in my medical texts, a series of events in my personal life were leading me to conclusions about the role diet plays in our health that frankly shocked me. What I discovered was eye opening—and as a result I was motivated to completely change my approach to medicine and break free from the status quo, setting me on a mission to spread this message of truth. I will not stop. It's too important, and people urgently need to hear this.

My personal path to better health

I'm the guy who always has a five- and a ten-year plan and believes that it's all going to come to fruition. But never in a million years did I think that I'd one day be an advocate for plant-based gut health. To understand why, you have to understand my background.

I was raised on the standard American diet. Nothing against my parents: I think this is how most kids were raised in the early '80s. It was normal in our house to eat Doritos and drink Purplesaurus Rex Kool-Aid every single day. Convenience reigned supreme. There were a lot of SpaghettiOs with Meatballs, Chef Boyardee Ravioli, and frozen burritos.

In high school, my parents were divorced and my mom worked full-time. My brothers and I would come home from school, fire up the propane grill, and have a few hot dogs. I became a hot dog connoisseur. Nathan's Famous and Hebrew National were the top brands, although if you could get your hands on the local Hofmann brand hot dogs, that was next level.

Now, before I go any further, I'd like to take a step back and honor my mom, who was an incredible parent and worked tirelessly to provide for our family. To her credit, she was pretty diligent about reminding us to eat more fruits and vegetables. Being the typical teenage boy, I not only rejected this notion but actually prided myself on pushing the limits of what my body was capable of consuming on the opposite end of the spectrum. I had that sense of invincibility that most of us have at that age. I felt like I could eat anything I wanted and was immune to any consequences.

My poor eating continued. My college diet at Vanderbilt was predominantly cold-cut sandwiches from Jersey Mike's and Jimmy John's with a late-night sprinkling of Wendy's, Sonic, and Waffle House. I started drinking massive quantities of soda to the point where it became a two-liter-per-day habit. During medical school at Georgetown I was obsessed with Wisemiller's Deli, which was a short walk from campus. These two subs were the ultimate back then:

Chicken madness: Mounds of grilled chicken breast, onions, sweet peppers, garlic, hot pepper, provolone cheese, bacon, lettuce, tomato, and mayonnaise. Wowza!

Burger madness: Two quarter pounders with American cheese, bacon, grilled onions, lettuce, tomato, and mayonnaise. Make sure the bathroom's close!

Honestly, it's incredible that I never had a heart attack. I had those two sandwiches at least three times a week.

This pattern of unapologetically eating poorly may seem cheeky or cute, but it was taking a toll on my body. As I became busier with work, took less time for exercise, and started to inch closer to age thirty, I began gaining weight, leaned heavily on coffee to get me through the day, and generally felt unwell.

Things came to a head during my year as chief medical resident at Northwestern. All of my dreams were coming true professionally. Beyond being selected as the chief medical resident, which is a huge honor, I had received all the other major awards in our residency program. I was already the author of eight scientific papers in the top gastroenterology journals and my mentors, two of the most famous GI doctors in the country, Drs. John Pandolfino and Peter Kahrilas, were touting me as the next great clinical investigator. Northwestern was paying all of my expenses so that I could get a master's degree in clinical research, which I was doing in night school in addition to all my other responsibilities.

Everything from the outside seemed like it was going great, like off the charts better than my wildest expectations. But on the inside I was miserable. I was completely exhausted, overworked, and the invincible feeling of my younger years was gone as my body started to change. My weight crept higher and higher until I was nearly fifty pounds overweight. I didn't like the way I looked or felt, but I was too busy to do anything about it.

It never crossed my mind that having dry-aged steaks at the Chicago chophouses twice a week with the hospital bigwigs or grabbing chili cheese dogs and Italian beef sandwiches on the way home wasn't doing me any good. I was a celebrated doctor at one of America's elite medical institutions, and I had such little awareness about nutrition that I was completely incapable of advising my patients, let alone myself. In hindsight, of course, it's obvious how unhealthy my diet was. It's not that I thought I was eating healthy. It's more that this was normal for me. I'd been eating this way for years, so why should I change things now?

The following year I moved to Chapel Hill for my gastroenterology fellowship at the University of North Carolina, the top GI division in the country. I stopped seeing patients for eighteen months and was completely immersed in the world of clinical research as a cancer epidemiologist. During this time I presented more than forty times at national meetings; I published more than twenty papers in the top peer-reviewed journals in my field; I was even selected to give the Presidential Plenary on the biggest stage at the biggest international

GI meeting of the year, Digestive Disease Week. With the help of my amazing mentor, Dr. Nick Shaheen, we were shifting paradigms.

While in Chapel Hill, I met my future wife, Valarie, and that's when things really changed. The way she ate was completely different from the way of anyone I'd ever met. We'd go out to dinner at a nice restaurant, and there'd be a menu filled with a myriad of steaks, chops, poultry, and seafood, but she would get the vegetable plate. Huh? I kept it to myself, but on the inside I had an eyebrow raised. Honestly, I didn't have any friends who were vegan or vegetarian. This was a mind-boggling experience for me.

But I couldn't contend with the results. Val ate without restriction. She never worried about portion size and yet never seemed to have issues controlling her weight. She was smoking hot! (And still is.) Meanwhile I was over here sweating out thirty-minute workouts plus a forty-five-minute run every day, and physically strong but still carrying far more weight than I was comfortable with. The way she ate made me curious, so I started to experiment at home without telling her. At first it was making big smoothies with kale and berries that I would do as a replacement for fast food. Immediately, I noticed that I didn't have that post-meal hangover where you're just completely exhausted for two or three hours. I loved the way I felt on those days—lighter, more energized, stronger. I also noticed changes with my body—glowing skin, thicker hair, thinner face. My clothes started to fit me differently. My mind had more stamina for work. My mood was lifted and optimistic.

I was feeling so good that I began to wonder why I'd never heard anything about the benefits of a plant-based diet in my medical training. My assumption was that there must not be any studies, that it must be empiricism. The advantage of having a master's degree in clinical investigation, doing an epidemiology fellowship at the number two school of public health, and publishing more than twenty scientific papers is that you don't need someone else to interpret the research for you. You do it yourself. So when I went to the medical literature, I was absolutely shocked by what I found. There was a *mountain* of evidence to support the way I was feeling. We're not talking a few bad studies where the truth was stretched or there were hyperbolic claims. I'm talking about study after study providing a uniform, consistent result. Plants are good for our health.

There's so much to love about eating plants. They're nutrient dense and calorie poor, the ideal weight-loss combination. They have vitamins, minerals, antioxidant compounds called polyphenols, and unique medicinal chemicals only found in plant food called phytonutrients. But there's one particular part of the plant that absolutely stole my heart—FIBER. Everything I thought I knew about fiber has been turned on its head, and I now legitimately believe that this is the single most important missing piece in the American diet. As you'll see in this book, this isn't your grandma's fiber. This is the true gut health game changer.

As time went on I continued to make changes in my own life. It wasn't an overnight or radical change. These were small choices over the course of time that were adding up—eliminating soda; cutting out fast food; adding in plant-based smoothies, soups, and salads. Exploring different flavors of ethnic foods that I hadn't tried before—Indian, Thai, Vietnamese, and Ethiopian. I'm drooling just thinking about them. As I was going through this exploratory phase and making these changes, my body was changing, too. I couldn't lose weight on hour-long workouts when I ate poorly, but I was now so busy both professionally and personally that I didn't have time for exercise and the weight was melting off. As I brought myself closer and closer to a fully plant-based diet, I saw progress and improvements in my health and body. I was pescatarian for several years, and when I gave up the fish, eggs, and dairy I lost another fifteen pounds within a few months. I wasn't restricting myself; I mean I was crushing some serious food—diving face-first into delicious plant-based meals and barely coming up for air. Meanwhile I was down to my college weight. Jeans that for several years I had to jump off the bed to fit into needed a belt. And the belt needed new holes. People were saying to me everywhere I went, "Have you lost weight?" I was getting older in years, but apparently younger in appearance because I increasingly was being questioned if I was really old enough to be a doctor.

When I (finally) went into practice for the first time after sixteen years as a trainee, I was armed with a clinical skill set that had garnered me the top awards in both residency and fellowship, elite research training that empowered me to interpret the studies myself, and the wholehearted belief based upon the studies I'd read and my own personal experience that diet and lifestyle were at the root of all health and disease. Add to that my innate drive to provide my patients with the best care regardless of the money or the rules, and what came from that is a formula that blends the best of Western medicine with a scientifically validated nutrition and lifestyle approach.

The most shocking part for me was how well it worked. I shouldn't have been so surprised, since I'd experienced the benefits firsthand and seen the powerful science in the studies. I truly believed that if I could have just one patient make these lifestyle changes, then I'd done more good than if I treated an entire month's worth of patients with medicine. But the crazy part is, *hundreds* of my patients were making lifestyle modifications. Even by just making small adjustments, they were seeing a difference. But the ones who made me truly excited were those who made radical changes. I was as excited as they were as I watched them transform into the healthy, vibrant people they had always wanted to be.

As I witnessed this happen time and again, I began to feel an increasing sense of urgency to share this message of plant-based gut health. It wasn't enough to share this story with my patients behind closed doors. Everyone deserved to hear this truth and to be given the opportunity to transform their life for the better. The world needs this healing!

I'd witnessed the confusion that the internet and so-called gut experts had created by promoting messages that were on trend but completely lacking any scientific basis. I'd seen far too many patients harm their bodies with the latest fad diet. These were well-intentioned people who were motivated to improve their health and willing to make lifestyle changes to make it happen. But unfortunately the advice they were being fed by the system was failing them. They were told, "Do this and you'll be better," only they weren't better. They were worse. The philosophy of "eliminate the symptoms by eliminating the food" was not only failing them, it was giving many of them an eating disorder. Some just orthorexia, but I've seen numerous cases of full-blown anorexia nervosa start with commitment to a restrictive diet. And as I watched, the entire popular conversation on gut health was building momentum yet missing the most important point—that it's the plants in your diet that fuel a healthy gut.

So I decided to create an Instagram account, which I titled @theguthealthmd, to share my message on a broader scale. Completely new to social media, I had no idea what to expect. Through word of mouth, a few podcast appearances, and a profile piece by our local newspaper, I began to get a steady stream of new followers to my account. Messages began pouring in from people all over the world, telling me about the improvements they were seeing in their lives through making the adjustments I recommended. I heard stories of people who were losing weight, able to come off medications, and feeling better than they had in years.

I soon realized that it wasn't enough. In order to give people the opportunity to really make lasting change and transform their lives, I needed to share the entire step-by-step plant-based gut health program that I was using with my patients in my clinic. That became the book you are holding in your hands right now.

I want to welcome you to the start of an exciting, transformative journey. I've seen the results from this program time and time again in my own patients, and now you can experience those results for yourself. As you follow this program, you will optimize your microbiome, eliminate cravings, strengthen your immune system, improve energy levels, and resolve digestive issues. This is not a fad or a diet; this is a lifestyle that empowers you to better health. With a "health mindset," you will effortlessly level up with healthy habits and your gut microbes will rejoice as they thrive on being *Fiber Fueled*.

To view the 4 scientific references cited in this chapter, please visit me online at www.theplantfedgut.com/research/.

PART I
KNOWLEDGE IS POWER

1

The Engine that Drives Human Health Isn't Even Human

You've got friends in low places—trillions of them!

When I graduated medical school in 2006, we knew next to nothing about the gut microbiota. At that time 60 percent of gut microbes did not grow on a traditional culture plate, so we really didn't have a way to study them. We knew they existed but didn't have a way to extract any intel on them. And honestly, we weren't losing any sleep over it. I mean, we're talking about the bacteria in our poop! Butt bugs! From our perspective, those scalawags were just along for the ride and not necessarily playing an important role in our health.

But things changed dramatically with a laboratory breakthrough in 2006 that moved us past the culture plate and allowed us to peel apart the complex layers of our gut microbiome and study them. Up to this point we only knew of about two hundred species of bacteria that inhabited the human gut. Very quickly, we identified fifteen thousand species and there are estimates now that there may be as many as thirty-six thousand. Our barrier to research had been removed and the floodgates opened. Since then there's been an absolute *explosion* of science, with 12,900 papers on the topic in the last five years alone. To put that number into perspective, this represents a full 80 percent of the papers on the topic in the last forty years.

Maybe you've heard something about the importance of the gut microbiome, but trust me, whatever you've read is just scratching the surface. All of this science is coming at us incredibly fast, and admittedly it is a challenge for our health care system to manage. It takes an average of seventeen years for new findings to go from publication to being in the clinic or in the consciousness of doctors, so most doctors are still functioning in the culture plate era. All have heard of the microbiome, but for most they haven't figured out how to include this information in their clinical practice. But why wait? I've monitored the emerging research with wide eyes and a gaping jaw and I'm ready to share it with you right now. No seventeen-year wait.

What we discovered when we learned to study gut bacteria is a shockingly broad, expansive community of microorganisms that live inside us in harmony, in balance, and with a purpose. We call this community the "gut microbiota." If we're referring specifically to the genetic code of this community, then we use the expression "microbiome." There are five types of microorganisms residing within you. They include bacteria, yeasts, parasites, viruses, and archaea.

Bacteria are living single-celled organisms that most of us grew up fearing. Believe it or not, our fears are strongly misplaced. Yes, there are some like *E. coli* or *Pseudomonas* that are bad and create issues for us. But most are actually good and are trying to help us. They're like dogs. Most are man's best friend, but some you'd rather not reach out to pet. For those, you need a dog whisperer. But if we're talking about the gut microbiota, then you need someone like me, the Poop Whisperer.

Fungi are multicellular organisms that, similar to animals and plants, have a nucleus and other organelles. They're more sophisticated than bacteria but, similar to bacteria, they are often thought to be bad even though many are trying to help us. They also compete with bacteria, which means that there's a zero-sum game: if one is flourishing, then the other is withering.

Viruses are tiny particles made up of DNA (or RNA) that don't have a cell at all and aren't even considered to be living, even though they share some qualities with us animate folk. Illnesses like influenza, HIV, and hepatitis B are often the first to come to mind when we think of viruses, but not all viruses are trying to hurt humans. In fact, most are an important part of the balanced gut microbial community and are necessary to keep our bacteria in harmony.

Parasites are nature's thieves. They steal energy from the host and try to remain undetected without offering any benefit. There are many types, ranging from giardia to the "trich" (pronounced "trick," a sexually transmitted infection) to the terrifying worms that can be up to eighty feet long and give me the heebie-jeebies. Thankfully, most parasites (such as those worms) are rare in the Western world, although there are some that are more common than you'd expect. For example, sixty million Americans are chronically infected with *Toxoplasma gondii* and don't know it because they are asymptomatic.

And then there's archaea, my personal favorite. These ancient organisms were on our planet before oxygen even existed four billion years ago, and you'll find them miles deep in the ocean in rift vents or inside a volcano. You'll also find them chilling in the friendly comforts of your colon. The point here is that these are *resilient* organisms. We're just starting to learn about them, but, for what it's worth, they don't seem to compete with the bacteria and fungi for energy so they don't appear to be manipulated by diet quite as easily as the other parts of our microbiota.

The depth of the gut microbiota is hard to fathom. It's like trying to wrap your mind around the Battle of Stalingrad in World War II where there were nearly two million casualties in a single battle. The numbers are so astronomical that you're forced to ignore that each one was an individual, a real person. In this case, we carry thirty-nine trillion microorganisms in our colons. Thirty-nine trillion! Most of them bacteria.

But don't feel ashamed or grossed out by that—I mean, okay, it is kind of gross, but I'm here to tell you that the bacteria in your gut and, as you'll soon see, in your bowel movements, too, are a wondrous, magical community with amazing healing power. After all, even Ryan Gosling has bacteria in his colon. How bad could they possibly be?

So how many microbes is thirty-nine trillion? Imagine you are up in the northern parts of Canada on a very clear night, and you can look up and see literally every single star in the Milky Way. Take that number of stars and multiply it by a hundred and that's how many microorganisms are in your colon. That number clearly outpaces the number of human cells in your body. Depending on how you look at it, some would say you are only 10 percent human—and 90 percent bacteria! You're not just human, you're a superorganism that serves as an ecosystem for four of the six kingdoms of life: Eubacteria, Fungi, Archaebacteria, and Protista. The other two are Animalia (us) and plantae (what we eat). We are more than *just* human. We are the circle of life.

The human gut is all interconnected in a way that draws direct comparisons to planet Earth. Your gut microbiome is just as much of an ecosystem as the Amazon rain forest. It thrives on balance and harmony. In the jungle, all animals, plants, and microbes exist with a purpose, even the mosquitoes and snakes. They all bring something to that harmonious balance, and as much as I hate mosquitoes and snakes, their loss would have unintended consequences and diminish the health of that ecosystem. This is why biodiversity is critically important to any ecosystem.

The human gut microbiome is no exception. Diversity of species is critically important to balance. Inside us are anywhere from three hundred to over a thousand species of bacteria (out of the fifteen thousand to thirty-six thousand in existence). When things are working the way they're supposed to, we have a diverse, abundant community of microbes living in harmony in our colon. The colon itself is healthy and strong with an intact barrier of cells to keep everything in its rightful place, and our microbiota plays its natural role as the workhorses of human health.

As residents of the intestines, it comes as no surprise that they are critically involved in digestive function. They work in teams to unpack your food, allowing you to extract the nutrients you need. There's not a meal that goes by that your microbes aren't busy at work helping you to break down your food and get the most out of it. It's hard to fathom, but in many cases these single-celled organisms are better at digesting our food than we are. As a result, we have evolved to rely on them for that.

Every single bite, all three pounds of food per day, flows downstream to your gut microbes. They are not passive observers. Our food is also their food. Yes, even invisible unicellular organisms need an energy source to fuel them. But not every microbe eats the same food. Each dietary choice you make will empower a specific group of microbes, while others will languish. If you permanently remove a food group, the microbes that thrive on that food will starve into extinction. They are procreating so quickly that the food choices you make in twenty-four hours will alter the evolution of fifty generations of microbes. It doesn't take days or even weeks to change your microbes; it only takes one bite. But you control what it is you bite into, and therefore you control the makeup of your microbiome.

The end result is a unique mix of microbes, as unique as a fingerprint. Those microbes go to work on your food and things don't end the way they started. Microbial metabolism leads to biochemical transformation of the food. In many cases, the healthy bacteria (let's call them probiotic) will reward us by molding our food into something that reduces inflammation and promotes health and balance. We call the health-promoting compounds created by our microbes postbiotics. But the opposite can also be true. Unhealthy food feeds unhealthy microbes, and they punish us by creating compounds that inflame our body. We'll be talking about a few of these, such as TMAO (trimethylamine N-oxide), in this book.

Anything that you put into your mouth will be processed by these microbes, including drugs. Which helps to explain why the same drugs can have a lifesaving effect in one person and a life-threatening effect in another. For example, the chemotherapy drug cyclophospha-mide actually depends on gut microbes to activate it. The healthier the gut, the better the chance at fighting off cancer with this drug, according to a 2013 study published in *Science*.

That's not the only thing we rely on them for. What's cool is that the health effects extend far beyond the walls of the colon. If I were to boldly define the entirety of human health, there would be five essential elements: immunity, metabolism, hormonal balance, cognition, and gene expression. That would cover our bases for everything we need to thrive as humans, and what's amazing is that the microbiota is intertwined with all five axes of human health. We're going to dive deeper into this, but let's start by acknowledging the gut microbiota as a command center of sorts for human health. Things happening throughout the body, the heart and brain included, often have their origins in the work of the gut microbes. They work as teams, but often with specialization.

Imagine the gut as a factory staffed by workers with many different roles. Each individual contributes his or her expertise toward the greater cause. And yes, there will be overlap in terms of expertise. If you lose Sally the engineer, but you replace her with Mark the engi-neer, you may find some differences in how they work but that their similar skill set allows them both to accomplish the required task. But if you lose an engineer and ask the conveyor belt operator to fill in, what's going to happen? Or what happens if instead of a range of spe-cialties like engineers, conveyor belt operators, woodworkers, welders, and technicians, you just had every position staffed by sales reps? That's when the factory stops functioning well, signals get crossed, and things break down. In the same way, when you lack diversity in your gut microbiome, mistakes happen in those five major areas: immunity, metabolism, hormones, cognition, and gene expression. It's all inter-connected, but at the heart of it is your gut microbiota.

We use the term "dysbiosis" to refer to the loss of harmony and balance within the gut. Damage or microbial disruption causes you to lose diversity and, in the process, see a higher proportion of inflammatory microbes emerge. In other words, the good stuff falls to the way-side, making more room for the not-so-good stuff to flood your gut. This is problematic because now the colon wall is no longer protected by a healthy community of anti-inflammatory bugs, and the result is damage to the tight junctions holding the colon wall together and an increase in intestinal permeability—some call this "leaky gut"—that leads to the spillage of something called bacterial endotoxin into the bloodstream. This bacterial endotoxin jumps on the vascular super-highway throughout the body, and wherever it goes, it sets a fire (better known as inflammation). It's bad news!

Bacterial endotoxin is produced by evildoer bacteria like *E. coli* and *Salmonella* and promotes inflammation that can range from smolder-ing and low-grade all the way up to life-threatening sepsis, shock, and multi-organ failure. Bacterial endotoxemia has been linked to a myriad of diseases including autoimmunity, obesity, coronary artery disease, congestive heart failure, type 2 diabetes, Alzheimer's, alco-holic hepatitis, nonalcoholic fatty liver, osteoarthritis . . . I could keep going.

Sounds terrifying, but don't be scared. The light always drowns out the darkness. Let me give you an example. There's a bacteria known as *Clostridiodes difficile*, formerly known as *Clostridium difficile* (yes, like Prince and Puff Daddy, apparently bacteria change their names, too), and often called *C. diff* for short. *C. diff* is a pathogenic bacteria that can exist in the colon, even in those who are healthy and living their best lives. In this setting, the healthy gut bacteria outnumber the troublesome *C. diff* and are able to suppress it. Light outshines the darkness.

But if the gut is damaged and there aren't enough good guys, *C. diff* multiplies, becomes stronger, and causes colitis (severe inflammation of the colon) with abdominal pain, fever, and explosive blood-drenched diarrhea. It's not pretty. This can progress to sepsis, a life-threatening response to infection that can rapidly take even the healthiest of lives. When this is the case, emergency surgery to remove the entire colon may be needed as a last-ditch effort to get the infection out and save the person's life.

When I was in medical school in the early 2000s, we *only* saw *C. diff* in hospitalized patients who were taking antibiotics. In retrospect we understand that napalming the gut with antibiotics decimates the good bacteria, allowing the antibiotic-resistant *C. diff* to rise up and dominate. Back then we didn't fully understand this, so we tried to treat the *C. diff* infection with, you guessed it, another antibiotic. This worked for a while, but by around 2010 we were seeing more and more cases of antibiotic failures. We also were seeing *C. diff* pop up in a new group—young people who had never been on antibiotics and had never been in the hospital. Things were changing so quickly that most of what I was taught in medical school was outdated just a few years later. As antibiotic effectiveness dwindled, we became increasingly desperate as a medical community. Some people were requiring long-term treatment with antibiotics, while the less fortunate were losing their colon or their life.

But remember, the light drowns out the darkness. So in our time of desperation, modern medicine turned to the most bizarre and humbling of places—human stool. That's not a typo, folks! Yes, we used poop as our treatment. It's called a fecal transplant, and it's not as novel as it may seem. The earliest reports are from ancient China more than fifteen hundred years ago. Turns out, when you transfer the fecal microbiota of a heathy person into the colon of an extremely sick person—or, in this specific example, when you douse the *C. diff* with healthy poop—this vicious, drug-resistant infection reacts like the Wicked Witch of the West after Dorothy threw the bucket of water on her. The *C. diff* cries, "I'm melting, I'm melting," and the person is cured—not just better, but *cured*—in one or two days. I told you, the light drowns out the darkness. I'd call it a miracle, except miracles aren't supposed to be reproducible.

So what is it about a fecal transplant that makes it so special? It's actually pretty simple: You are restoring balance to the gut microbiota. You're putting the right bacteria back to work in the factory. When you do that, they do their job and immediately dominate and suppress the pathogenic *C. diff,* just like we previously described happens in someone who is colonized but doesn't have the infection.

"But isn't my stool just waste from food digestion?" you may be asking. Nope. Sixty percent of the weight of your stool is actually bacteria, both good and bad. Sixty percent! It's a snapshot of what your gut microbiota looks like. Not a perfect snapshot, but it's essentially a blend of bacteria from throughout the colon. Even if you fast, you'd still produce stool because your gut microbiota is constantly replicating and turning over.

We all love a feel-good story, right? The comeback of the century, the millennium even, is our stool. What was the least valuable thing on the planet ten years ago has become the savior of modern medicine. People say, "Food is medicine." It's true, but "Poop is medicine, too!" For generation after generation we disparaged it with poop jokes when we should have been celebrating it, or at least giving it a respectful tip of the cap. We didn't realize that our stool was the chariot carrying our celebrated gladiator, the gut microbiota. I'm not exaggerating; I sincerely believe our bowel movements should be the sixth vital sign. Body temperature, pulse, respiratory rate, blood pressure, oxygen saturation, and last (but not least) bowel movement quality. It really is a powerful window into our health.

My point here is that balance is absolutely critical to the gut flora and to every part of your body that operates in communication with it. All those years that we were trying to destroy the bad guys, all we needed to do was empower the good guys. When that balance is in place, your gut microbiota is really, really good at taking care of you. So powerful are the organisms in your gut that even in their "waste" form they can heal someone who's deathly ill.

There's no need to live in fear of the darkness when this book will help you create the light. Rather than trying to destroy the bad guys, let's work together to empower the good guys, restore balance to our command center, and allow the thirty-nine trillion workhorses to naturally enhance our immune system, metabolism, hormonal balance, cognition, and gene expression.

The awesome power of our gut microbiota for total body health

A healthy, diverse gut microbiome does so much more than just suppress pathogenic bacteria, process our drugs, and help us to process our food. It operates as the command center for all five axes of human health. It's bordering on science fiction, but it's absolutely true. I totally believe that all health and disease starts in the gut. The awe-inspiring power in our microbiota makes me reconsider my place on this planet. We, too, are a part of nature's balance, and inside us is this community that we need just as much as it needs us—we're better together! And when we take care of them, they take care of us.

SYMPTOMS ASSOCIATED WITH DAMAGE TO THE GUT MICROBIOTA (DYSBIOSIS)	
INTESTINAL	EXTRAINTESTINAL
Abdominal pain or cramping	Weight gain
Gas	Fatigue
Bloating/abdominal distension	Brain fog
Food sensitivities	Difficulty concentrating
Food allergies	Mood imbalance
Diarrhea	Anxiousness
Constipation	Skin breakouts
Mucus in stool	Joint pains or muscle aches
Nausea	Weakness
Indigestion	Bad breath
Heartburn/reflux	Sinus congestion
Belching	Shortness of breath/wheezing

Insights into the immune system from a toddler's diaper

While most of us are stunned by the emergence of human waste as actual medicine, someone who would probably not be so surprised by this revelation is Professor David Strachan, an epidemiologist at the London School of Hygiene and Tropical Medicine. In 1989 Strachan proposed the hygiene hypothesis upon observing that infants born into a household with more siblings were less susceptible to eczema and allergic rhinitis. You may have heard of his hypothesis—it's the theory that excessive cleanliness is behind the explosion of allergic and autoimmune disease. It's why some families encourage their kids to play in the dirt to benefit their immunity!

Professor Strachan's observations were a good start. But modern science is now showing us that we need to take it a step further. The true problem is not so much excessive cleanliness as it is damage and disruption of the healthy gut microbiota. As I mentioned, a full 70 percent of the immune system lives in the gut, separated from our microbiota by a single layer of cells that is a fraction of the diameter of a hair and undetectable by the human eye. That single layer of cells acts like a three-foot rickety wooden fence between two house parties—with the immune system at one house and the microbiota at the other. The parties may be separate, but they're not *really* separated. They're deeply intertwined, feeding off each other's energy, sharing drinks and laughs, in constant communication with one another. Evidence has shown us that the microbiota helps foster proper development of immune cells, identify invaders, get immune cells to the needed location, and then enhance their infection-fighting power. A healthy gut microbiota translates into an empowered, strong immune system that optimally functions to identify a threat when it exists— infectious or even malignant—and eradicate it. You can't separate the gut microbiota from the immune system. If you hurt one, you will hurt the other.

Evidence for the gut-immune relationship comes from the autoimmune and allergic epidemic. These conditions are indeed exploding around the world. Asthma, allergic rhinitis, and eczema are examples of allergic diseases, where the immune system aggressively attacks a benign outside stimulus. From 1960 to 2000 the incidence of asthma increased at least tenfold in the Western world. A similar, disturbing rise in autoimmune diseases has occurred in parallel. Type 1 diabetes, multiple sclerosis, and Crohn's disease are autoimmune diseases, where the immune system decides our own body is the enemy and goes on the attack. Since the 1950s, the rates of type 1 diabetes, multiple sclerosis, and Crohn's disease have each risen 300 percent or more.

Allergic and autoimmune conditions are much more common in industrialized nations than in agricultural ones. For example, the number of new cases of type 1 diabetes in Finland per year is 62.3 per every 100,000 children, compared with just 6.2 in Mexico and 0.5 in Pakistan. You could argue that that's due to genetic differences, but they also appear to increase in prevalence within countries as they become more industrialized. Croatia, for example, has seen an increase in Crohn's disease from 0.7 per 100,000 (in 1989) to 6.5 (in 2004), coinciding with modernization, and Brazil saw Crohn's disease and ulcerative colitis increase by 11 and 15 percent *every year* from 1988 to 2012, respectively. Doctors from these countries have to come to the United States to learn about these conditions because the problems didn't exist in their countries until recently, so they don't know how to care for their patients.

Evidence suggests that our gut microbiome not only changes with allergic and autoimmune disease, but it may predict or even cause these immune system conditions. For example, researchers analyzed the dirty diapers of three hundred toddlers at three months of age. They discovered that specific changes in the gut bacteria this early in life already predicted which children would subsequently develop asthma years later. But to prove that the gut microbes were actually causing the asthma, they transferred the stool from the diapers into special germ-free mice. Yes, they did a fecal transplant from a human into a mouse. And to be clear, the human stool wasn't from a person with asthma. Instead, it was from a three-month-old's poopy diaper who was felt to be at risk for developing asthma. So what happened? Well, the mice all developed inflamed lungs, indicative of asthma.

We evolved to have an immune system to protect us from infection, the leading cause of death up until just a century ago. Our gut microbes have been a part of that evolution from the very beginning, and as a result they play a critical role in immune function. Yes, this can mean that damage to the microbiota puts us at risk for immune dysregulation, manifesting with autoimmune and allergic illness. But on the flip side, a strong microbiome empowers the 70 percent of neighboring immune cells for optimal function to protect us from infection and malignancy. When we take care of our microbes, they take care of us.

IMMUNE-MEDIATED CONDITIONS ASSOCIATED WITH DYSBIOSIS	
Type 1 diabetes mellitus	Rheumatoid arthritis
Celiac disease	Ulcerative colitis
Multiple sclerosis	Crohn's disease
Asthma	Microscopic colitis
Food allergies	Ankylosing spondylitis
Eczema	Lupus
Seasonal allergies	Interstitial cystitis
Eosinophilic esophagitis	Autoimmune hepatitis
Dermatitis herpetiformis	Primary biliary cholangitis
Psoriasis/psoriatic arthritis	Primary sclerosing cholangitis
Scleroderma	Sarcoidosis
Chronic fatigue syndrome	Fibromyalgia
Antiphospholipid syndrome	Guillain-Barré syndrome
Restless leg syndrome	Behçet's disease
Sjögren's syndrome	Kawasaki disease
	ANCA-associated vasculitis

The Microbiome Code for personalized food processing

The diet industry has for a very long time told us that weight gain is within our control if we could only have the self-control to do enough CrossFit/Zumba/yoga in combination with the right diet, whether that's Paleo, SlimFast, Weight Watchers, Keto, or juice cleanses. But what if it all comes down to the bacteria in our guts? That's what researchers recently set out to discover when a report emerged of a young woman, just thirty-two years old, who underwent a fecal transplant for a chronic *C. diff* infection. What ensued got both scientists and the press into a tizzy. In the sixteen months after her fecal transplant she had dramatic, unintentional weight gain—going from 136 pounds up to 170 pounds. Her body mass index increased from very nearly a normal, healthy weight (BMI of 26) up to overt obesity (BMI of 33). Nothing else in her life had changed: not her diet, not her stress level, not her level of physical activity. Just the fecal transplant.

Normally weight gain of this kind wouldn't be such a big deal except that for the first time in humans we had illustrated an idea that has been shown repeatedly, time after time, in animals: that our gut microbiota has extreme control over the way that we process our food and our metabolism. So much control, in fact, that the same food can yield totally different effects depending on the gut microbiota involved.

One study took identical human twins who were genetically the same but one was obese and the other thin. Researchers took stool from the twins and transferred it into germ-free mice, and the mouse that got the lean twin's stool stayed lean and the one who got the obese twin's became obese. Despite the fact that both mice were fed the exact same diet and exact same calories, they found that the body type transferred.

So many of us have spent years working really hard to lose weight—exercising, eating well, doing all the things experts (and the not-so-expert) are telling us to do—and now we understand why that might not be working. We need a little help from our friends. You can give the exact same food to two different people and the differences in their microbiota will determine what they ultimately get out of that food. Mind blowing, isn't it?

But it doesn't stop there. Our microbiota doesn't just regulate our metabolism in a calories-in, calories-out sense. It is also deeply intertwined with our endocrine system, affecting our response to insulin. After a meal your blood sugar level rises and the cells in your pancreas respond by releasing insulin into your bloodstream to lower your blood sugar. If you have diabetes, you have an inadequate supply of insulin to control your blood sugar, so it stays elevated. Type 1 diabetics have an autoimmune disease that destroys the part of their pancreas that produces insulin. As we discussed before, autoimmune type 1 diabetes connects back to gut health. On the flip side, type 2 diabetics have a fully functioning pancreas running on overdrive but they are unable to produce enough insulin to keep up with the body's demands. This is a result of insulin resistance, meaning more insulin has to be produced to achieve the same effect. Insulin is a growth factor. What do you think happens when you promote increased growth in the body? Type 2 diabetes has been linked to esophageal, colorectal, pancreatic, hepatocellular, renal, breast, endometrial, and urinary cancer.

Cancer stinks. Literally.

Did you know that dogs can actually smell colorectal cancer? They were 98 percent accurate in detecting colon cancer from a series of stool specimens. And you thought they were just sniffing backsides for fun? Give man's best friend some credit! Colorectal cancer is the number two cause of cancer death in America, and emerging studies are showing that specific bacteria in the colon play a role in its development, which may explain how they're able to do this. Alterations in gut bacteria have been associated with a number of emerging cancers: breast, gastric, esophageal, pancreatic, laryngeal, liver, and gallbladder carcinomas. Ongoing research is being performed to determine the degree for which the bacteria are actually causative.

We've already shown that your gut bacteria differentially regulate your response to food and can affect weight gain. How about your body's response to insulin? In an absolutely fascinating study, adult men with metabolic syndrome and insulin resistance received a fecal transplant from a lean donor. This led to a change in their gut microbiota associated with improvements in insulin sensitivity and a lowering of their blood sugar. Unfortunately, the effect only lasted a few weeks because they didn't change their diet, so the new microbiome couldn't be sustained.

But you don't need to have diabetes to show an influence from your

METABOLIC CONDITIONS ASSOCIATED WITH DYSBIOSIS	
Obesity	Nonalcoholic fatty liver disease
Type 2 diabetes	Alcoholic steatohepatitis
Coronary artery disease	Acute alcoholic hepatitis
Hyperlipidemia	Alcoholic cirrhosis
Chronic kidney disease	Acute pancreatitis
Gout	Chronic pancreatitis

gut microbiota! In another study, researchers discovered that foods had a very different blood sugar response in each person. The gut microbiome was responsible for this unique response. Using solely an individual's gut microbial profile, they were able to predict which foods would cause less of a blood sugar spike. It was different for every person. In other words, you have a unique, completely personal response to the food you eat that is a reflection of the makeup of your gut microbiota. Good ole bio-individuality, my friends!

Discard all (or most) of what you've ever learned about metabolism, diabetes, and weight loss. It's a loss of diversity in the gut microbiota, increase in pathogenic bacteria, and low-grade inflammation from bacterial endotoxin that is associated with diabetes, weight gain, and obesity. There is also evidence to suggest that our gut microbes control the release of hormones that regulate appetite and energy balance, such as leptin, ghrelin, GLP-1 (glucagon-like peptide-1), and peptide YY. Increased microbial diversity in your gut equals improved metabolic health and insulin sensitivity.

So when we properly nourish our gut microbiota, we are rewarded with microbes that extract everything that we need from our food and nothing that we don't, signal us when to stop eating so we don't overdo it, and promote a natural metabolic balance that doesn't require us to count calories in order to maintain a healthy weight. A healthy microbiome makes it happen effortlessly.

It's not your fault you're hormonal!

The influence of the gut microbiota on the endocrine, or hormonal, system extends far beyond diabetes. The gut is literally the largest endocrine organ in the body, deeply involved in securing hormonal balance. Take estrogen, for example. Gut microbes secrete the enzyme β-glucuronidase, which activates estrogen so it can do what it's supposed to do throughout the body. Imagine the flow of estrogen as a dammed river, and the microbes have their hand on a lever that controls the floodgates. When working just right, estrogen levels are delicately flowing in that sweet spot—not too much, not too little—to give the good stuff: stronger bones, lower cholesterol, clear skin, fertile ovaries, and a voracious sexual appetite. A healthy gut microbiota does that for you.

But what happens if you're loose on the floodgate? The body gets flooded with excess estrogen, which has been associated with endometriosis, endometrial hyperplasia, and breast and endometrial cancer. No surprise, we find damage to the gut microbiome in association with each of these conditions.

Alternatively, if the microbiota are too restrictive on the floodgates, you get an estrogen drought. Polycystic ovary syndrome (PCOS), which is characterized by menstrual irregularity, abnormal hair growth, weight gain, acne, and insulin resistance, is a condition that is characterized by estrogen dysregulation. But PCOS is a true loss of hormonal balance where there is an increase in androgens (or testosterone) in addition to altered estrogen. As it turns out, androgen production is also mediated in part by the gut microbiome. *Clostridium scindens* is a gut bacteria known to convert glucocorticoids (think cortisol) into androgens in the gut. So if you have too much *C. scindens* you'll have androgen excess. A healthy gut microbiome keeps our estrogens and androgens in balance, while dysbiosis has been found in association with PCOS.

It's quite clear that there's a gut-hormone axis, but let's take it a step further. It appears that there may be a gut-testicle axis, too. Fellas, listen up! Remember the model for dysbiosis? Damage to the gut microbiota causes increased intestinal permeability (leaky gut) and allows release of bacterial endotoxin into our system. Well, bacterial endotoxin leaves the gut and travels through the blood to the testicles, where it wreaks havoc. Science says it causes loss of testosterone and sperm production. It's kind of like gut health–induced "shrinkage." (Sorry for that mental image.) Not to mention the impact on mental health, which often includes loss of self-esteem and confidence.

But the link between gut health and hormones doesn't stop there. Have you ever been on a date and found yourself either super attracted to or turned off by your date based upon their smell? It's been demonstrated in animal studies that bacteria control the release of guaiacol and other phenolic compounds that produce our odor profile. These are actually pheromones that play a role in sexual attraction and mating behavior. In other words, our microbes are actually our matchmakers in waiting. What's interesting is that different microbes release different smells. The healthy microbes produce a fragrance worthy of Aphrodite, while the pathogenic bacteria drop a stench bomb that keeps people at their distance. Not every microbe makes a great wingman!

And while we're on the topic, have you ever wondered why we kiss? It's actually an expression of love to share your microbiome with another person. Every time we kiss we exchange eighty million microbes with our partner, and vice versa. There is speculation that kissing may have evolved as a way of sampling a potential lover's microbiome for compatibility. Yes, we are human. But everything that we do as humans involves our microbiota one way or another, even the way we love one another.

ENDOCRINE AND HORMONAL CONDITIONS ASSOCIATED WITH DYSBIOSIS	
Endometriosis	Hypothyroid
Polycystic ovary syndrome (PCOS)	Breast cancer
Endometrial hyperplasia	Endometrial cancer
Female infertility	Prostate cancer
Sexual dysfunction	Erectile dysfunction

The second brain's power over the first brain

Upstairs is your brain. Downstairs is your gut. Most would think of these organs as two very separate entities, with the brain operating as central command and the gut as what, well, makes you poop. In the hierarchy of things, clearly the brain would come out on top. But recently that line of division has become a bit blurred because we've discovered that the gut is a separate nervous system known as the "second brain" or the "enteric nervous system."

This might be the first time you're making this connection, but brain health actually starts in the gut—and that's because they are in constant communication with each other. Literally right this second, there are over five hundred million nerves in your intestines sending feedback to your brain through the vagus nerve. That's five times more nerves than you'll find in your spinal cord. That is a lot of information!

That's only the beginning. Gut microbes are able to communicate with our brain using the immune system and through the release of neurotransmitters, hormones, and signaling molecules. Neurotransmitters like serotonin and dopamine play a powerful role in our mood, energy levels, motivation, and sense of reward. Gut microbes both produce and respond to neurohormones like serotonin, dopamine, GABA (γ-aminobutyric acid), and norepinephrine. In fact, 90 percent of serotonin and 50 percent of dopamine are actually produced in the gut. Precursors of serotonin and dopamine are able to cross the blood–brain barrier and alter our mood or behavior. Taken in sum, intestinal serotonin is able to influence gut motility, mood, appetite, sleep, and brain function.

That's just serotonin. Your gut produces more than thirty neurotransmitters. In Chapter 3 we will discuss one of the major ways that your gut can improve brain health—through short-chain fatty acids. A healthy gut microbiome is able to extend its influence across the blood–brain barrier to keep our mind sharp, our energy level high, and our mood relaxed. But on the flip side, damage to the gut microbiome has been associated with Alzheimer's, Parkinson's, migraine headaches, chronic fatigue, autism, and ADHD.

With the gut acting as home base for these neurotransmitters, you can see how mental health conditions like depression and anxiety emerge when there's a problem in the gut. I see it every day in my clinic. For instance, there is tremendous overlap between irritable bowel syndrome (IBS) and depressed mood and anxiety. And for the longest time, we mislabeled these patients. We did not understand that at the root of their anxiety or vicious mood swings could be a gastrointestinal issue. It's now clear that when you have alteration or damage to the gut bacteria, you alter serotonin balance, and thereby alter both mood and gut motility. The end result is an IBS patient with anxiety. One of my mentors, Dr. Douglas Drossman, has for decades been at the center of the research to clarify this important connection.

We've also learned that IBS patients have altered function of the five hundred million gut nerves. It's what we call "visceral hypersensitivity," meaning that they will have intestinal distress, nausea, or abdominal pain in response to triggers that most people don't even notice. For example, IBS patients often *think* they produce more gas, but they actually don't. Instead, they produce the same amount of gas but they just react to it differently—due to increased visceral hypersensitivity.

Even our behavior is influenced by our gut. There is evidence to suggest that gut microbes control our cravings. Have you ever gone away on vacation for a few days and can't wait to get home and have one of your old stalwart meals? That's your microbiome speaking to you. In fact, gut microbes may put their well-being over ours by manipulating our eating behavior—some of them want us to eat sugar and fat, which are bad for us but good for them! They can promote their fitness at the expense of ours. You know how some people love chocolate (slowly raises hand) and others can take it or leave it? Well, we've found that "chocolate-desiring" people actually have different microbial metabolites in their urine than do "chocolate-indifferent" individuals, despite eating identical diets. Those microbial metabolites may be the signal that drives you to crave chocolate, which begs the question: Are we merely zombies, doing the will of our bacterial overlords? Are we pseudo-possessed by the bacterial demons in our gut? MUAAAHAAAHAAA!

Okay, now that I've got you all bug-eyed and freaked out, let's keep in mind that you are a creature of free will. Remember, you get to choose what you put in your mouth and swallow, and those choices are what will ultimately determine health in our microbiome and throughout our body. More important, your cravings and taste buds can change and you can train your gut to fall in love with things that are actually good for you. Following the plan in this book will allow you to break free once and for all—it's as though we're performing an exorcism from your gremlin-gut microbes and replacing them with guardian-gut angels.

NEUROPSYCHIATRIC CONDITIONS ASSOCIATED WITH DYSBIOSIS	
Alzheimer's disease	Anxiety
Parkinson's disease	Depression
Schizophrenia	Autism spectrum disorders
ADHD	Bipolar disorder
Amyotrophic lateral sclerosis	Migraine headaches
Chronic fatigue syndrome	Fibromyalgia
Restless legs syndrome	Hepatic encephalopathy

How the genetic game was turned on its head by microbes

Since 1953 when Professors James Watson and Francis Crick described the structure of DNA, it seemed that genetics held the keys to understanding human health and disease. Nearly fifty years later and after a massive coordinated international effort among one thousand scientists across twenty institutions, the Human Genome Project culminated in 2000 when the human genetic code was unlocked for the first time. This was as big as it gets from a scientific perspective.

Sadly, for all the hype, the returns on this breakthrough have been incredibly disappointing. You've no doubt noticed that we have not resolved all medical problems since the year 2000. Why did genetics alone not heal us? Well, we have since discovered by studying identical twins that less than 20 percent of disease is based on genetics. Yes, there are some, such as cystic fibrosis and Down syndrome, where if you have the genes then you get the disease. But taking all chronic disease across the board, more than 80 percent of your disease risk is determined by your environment and exposures during your lifetime. There's a silver lining here. You are not the victim of the genes you were born with. You may have certain predispositions—we all do. But you ultimately control your health destiny, in large part through the effects of your diet and lifestyle on your microbiome.

In a letter to *Science* magazine in 2001, Professor Julian Davies warned that decoding the human genome was not enough to understand human biology because there are more than a thousand bacterial species living in and on the human body and they are critically affecting human life. We previously noted that there are more bacteria than cells in the body, but let's take it a step further and talk genetics. More than 99 percent of your DNA comes from microbes. Yes, your genes are less than 1 percent human! Further, our human genomes are virtually identical—up to 99.9 percent the same. But our microbiomes may be as much as 90 percent *different* from one person to the next.

Beyond holding the cards on a genetic monopoly, our gut microbes also exert tremendous power over the expression of your genes through something called epigenetics. Imagine your gut microbiota as controlling a light switch and the wiring behind the wall is your genetic code. The gut microbiota is not changing the wiring behind the wall, but it can turn the lights on or off. You can't change your genetic code, but you can effect which genes get turned on or off. That is insanely powerful, if you think about it.

An example of this concept of epigenetics is celiac disease. Celiac disease is a condition in which the immune system decides that gluten is the enemy. Gluten is a protein found in wheat, barley, and rye. Every time someone with celiac disease consumes gluten, the immune system lashes out and attacks their intestine, causing inflammation that shows up as diarrhea, weight loss, and abdominal pain. This is incredibly dangerous because people with celiac disease who continue to consume gluten can develop small intestine lymphoma, which is nearly universally fatal.

Celiac is a genetically motivated disease. This means that you must carry the gene for celiac to get it. If you don't have the gene, you can't have the disease. About 35 percent of Americans carry the gene for celiac but only 1 percent manifest the disease. In the last fifty years we've seen a 500 percent increase in celiac disease. So what explains the rapid increase? Clearly not a shift in genetics during that brief period. So what is it that determines who ultimately expresses the gene? Dr. Elena Verdú from McMaster University in Canada showed us through a series of eloquent studies that there are three criteria that must be met to develop celiac disease: 1) presence of the gene, 2) exposure to gluten, and—you guessed it, 3) alteration or damage to the gut microbiota.

We thought that cracking the human genome would produce major breakthroughs in medicine because we thought that human health was primarily determined by genetic makeup. Nope. We are a superorganism with a genetic makeup dominated by the invisible microbes within us. And this is actually a good thing! Rather than worrying about the 0.5 percent of your DNA that you simply cannot control, let's optimize our microbiome through diet and lifestyle and enjoy the positive effects it has on 99.5 percent of our DNA plus our epigenetic expression.

It's time to transform your health from the inside out!

What once was dismissed as poop is now the star quarterback for human health. Yes, it can be intimidating that most modern diseases have been connected to damage to the gut microbiome. But remember, we are not helpless victims stricken with disease. We have the power of science on our side, and for the first time in human history we actually know enough about the gut microbiota to understand it and start to use it to our advantage. In this book I will use diet and lifestyle to rebalance your gut microbes. You'll see your digestion, immune system, metabolism, hormones, cognition, and gene expression become optimally aligned, and you'll transform into the microbe-empowered superhuman that you are.

To view the 55+ scientific references cited in this chapter, please visit me online at www.theplantfedgut.com/research/.

2

Twenty-First-Century Life: Overfed, Undernourished, and Hyper-medicated

Our modern lifestyle is destroying our gut AND our health

When I first met Kristen she sat with her shoulders slumped and her brow creased with worry. She came in to see me, hoping I'd address the chronic abdominal pain and diarrhea she'd been struggling with for years, but when I asked her to tell me more about what was going on, she launched into a litany of other concerns: "I feel sick all the time, Dr. B. I'm overweight, anxious, and depressed. I've got migraines and seasonal allergies so bad that I sometimes take antibiotics three or four times a year for sinus infections. I was also recently diagnosed with polycystic ovary syndrome." She took a deep breath. "And that really scares me." She told me about the slew of medications her various doctors had her on, and that she thought she may have sensitivity to gluten and beans and has eliminated them as part of doing the Paleo diet. Unfortunately, she wasn't feeling better so she was thinking about trying the Keto diet because she had several friends doing it and they were losing weight.

Kristen needs a plan that actually works. She knows she wants to fix her gut, but the approach of "eliminate symptoms by eliminating the foods that cause symptoms" hasn't worked for her. After multiple experts villainizing their poisons du jour—gluten, grains, phytates, lectins, carbs—Kristen misses the feeling of simply enjoying a meal. She wants to eat food that she loves, eat it in abundance and without restrictions, and not be constantly running away from food monsters. The good news for Kristen and everyone reading this is that I know exactly what you need to heal your gut.

Patients like Kristen are incredibly common in my gastroenterology clinic. Every day I meet people with stories like hers: people with complex medical problems, even at a very young age, coming to my clinic with digestive issues like irritable bowel syndrome (IBS), acid reflux, chronic diarrhea, abdominal pain, gas and bloating, or constipation. Often several at once. And what's shocking is how many *also* have immune-mediated disorders like type 1 diabetes, celiac, multiple sclerosis, Crohn's disease, ulcerative colitis, or rheumatoid arthritis, and are often coping with depression and anxiety, hormone imbalances, and weight gain, too.

It's not just in my clinic—nationwide, the statistics back this up. As a country we are fatter, sicker, and more heavily medicated than at any other time in human history. More than 72 percent of Americans are overweight—that's essentially three in four people—and 40 percent of us are carrying thirty or more pounds of extra baggage around our waist and hips. For the first time in over a hundred years, the U.S. life expectancy just dropped for the third year in a row. The last time this happened was from 1915 to 1918—when U.S. involvement in World War I and literally the worst influenza pandemic in modern history combined to kill nearly one million Americans. Last I checked we weren't conscripting an army for global battle or ravaged by a plague, so what's our excuse?

Despite advances in medicine and our spending more money on health care than any country in the world by far, our life expectancy is actually contracting. And now 60 percent of Americans age twenty or older are using prescription drugs. In fact, the percentage of us using five or more medications has doubled in the last twelve years. Yes, modern medicine has given us some wonderful treatment options—believe me, if I get sick, I want one of my esteemed colleagues caring for me—but we can't ignore the downsides of our love for quick-fix pills and overreliance on medications. Consider that in 2014 alone, nearly 1.3 million Americans sought emergency room treatment for adverse drug effects, and about 124,000 people died from them.

For me, and I'm guessing for you, too, since you picked up this book, these aren't just numbers on a page. Behind the numbers are real people—people like Kristen, who need more than another diagnosis, an additional script to fill, or yet another fad diet to follow based on bad science. If you're struggling with digestive issues, autoimmune illnesses, mental health, heart health, hormonal imbalance, weight gain, diabetes, or any related concerns, including side effects from taking several medications, I hear you and I see you. Many, many people sit across from me day after day in my clinic, often with tears in their eyes, who are struggling, too, and who need real help now. I have a fire in my heart to find the solution for these ailments that goes beyond a patch on the hole. We need to get at the root cause to reverse these diseases and prevent new ones.

The trend in our life expectancy isn't bad luck or a mere coincidence. Did you know that at least seven of the top ten causes of death—the things that are lowering our life expectancy—are caused by lifestyle? In order, they are: heart disease, cancer, chronic obstructive pulmonary disease (COPD), stroke, Alzheimer's, diabetes, and kidney disease. The problem is caused by lifestyle and yet we completely (and inexplicably) ignore lifestyle as a therapeutic option, choosing medications as our primary treatment option. By ignoring the cause we will never get to the root of the problem.

Sadly, the pharmaceutical industry has hijacked our health care system. Big Pharma runs the studies, they control the research, and here we are with three in five U.S. adults taking prescription drugs, 269 million prescriptions for antibiotics per year, 115 million proton pump inhibitor prescriptions, and 30 billion doses of nonsteroidal anti-inflammatory drugs (NSAIDs) like ibuprofen and naproxen. Meanwhile, obesity, and all the health issues that stem from it, seems to be becoming the new normal. On so many levels—our health, our food, even how often we poop—we are normalizing abnormal.

A medication treats symptoms. It artificially props up something that's broken. It doesn't prevent and it certainly doesn't treat root causes. It's time for us to stop waiting for the bomb to drop when our health deteriorates and we desperately need "sick care," and instead embrace true "health care" by preventing our problems with lifestyle medicine.

So when patients like Kristen come to me with a long list of symptoms, asking, "Doctor, why is this happening to me?" I don't just see the digestive issues they've come to me for; I see a web of interconnected symptoms. I see digestive concerns intertwined among multiple systems within the body: gynecologic, endocrine, neurologic, the immune system, even mood. And I know that the answer isn't cutting out gluten or beans or simply adding an additional medication for IBS—those are just covering up symptoms. The answer is at the root of it all—the place where it's all connected is in the gut.

Modernization and the origins of modern epidemics

In the late nineteenth century the average life expectancy was just forty-seven years and the top causes of death were infections. Infectious diseases such as smallpox, cholera, diphtheria, pneumonia, typhoid fever, tuberculosis, typhus, and syphilis were rampant. Heart disease and cancer were there, but a small problem compared to infections. Thanks to Louis Pasteur's discovery of what we now call modern germ theory, we finally understood that behind the top causes of death is a germ. In response, bacteria became public enemy numbers one, two, and three. So what are you going to do about it? Well, we did what humans have always done at every stage of human history—we innovated to find a solution to the problem in front of us. As we entered the twentieth century we started adding chlorine to our drinking water, developed vaccines, improved sanitation, and began metal canning and early preservatives. Good news, it was working: polio was on the brink of extinction, and many other infectious diseases, including smallpox, were on the decline. Then penicillin was discovered by Sir Alexander Fleming in 1928 and it became commercially available in 1945. Our life expectancy rapidly jumped over the coming years, and in 1969, U.S. Surgeon General William Stewart confidently declared to Congress that it was time to "close the books on infectious diseases."

Anything that good is going to get overutilized. We doubled down on this approach. In 1928 women were encouraged to "disinfect" with Lysol douche—yes, the same Lysol that today is used to scour toilets and floors. After World War II, we developed synthetic herbicides, fungicides, and insecticides. We added fluoride to the water. We discovered that antibiotics and synthetic hormones accelerated livestock growth, so we started pumping our livestock with both. We created antibacterial soaps and astringents and industrial cleaning products. If bacteria were the enemy, we were basically nuking the crap out of them. There's no question: We were winning this war.

And then heart disease and cancer emerged en masse.

Meanwhile, technology was developing on all fronts, for better or for worse. The number of food additives skyrocketed to more than ten thousand, the vast majority of which had never had human testing because they got approved under a loophole called GRAS (Generally Recognized As Safe, pronounced *GEE rass*). Remember this acronym—GRAS—because I'm coming back to it in a minute. Additionally, the pharmaceutical industry exploded and now more than fifteen hundred drugs were approved by the FDA, which explains why there was no nutrition training in medical school—we were spending all of our time learning about these drugs, their uses, and their side effects. Plastics, which contain bisphenol A (BPA), known to have estrogen-like effects, were invented and began to be used abundantly—in everything from food storage to floss and from clothing to baby toys. We developed planes, trains, automobiles, and motorized scooters to reduce our mobility. Advances in television, computers, smartphones, and video games made it easy to forgo exercise and hijack our brains and our daily sleep-wake cycles. Why read a book when watching the movie only takes ninety minutes? Why build a fort and imagine a game when a video game will do all the creative heavy lifting for you? Why go to sleep when the sun goes down when you can read Twitter all night long?

In 1994, genetically modified organisms (GMOs) first arrived in our stores. Today more than 80 percent of all genetically modified crops grown worldwide have been engineered to be herbicide tolerant. What this means is that the genetically modified plant survives being sprayed with herbicides while the surrounding plants (and potentially other life) all die. For example, Monsanto, the leading developer of GMOs, created a range of crops with a genetic trait that makes them impervious to the herbicide glyphosate, specifically soy beans and corn. We need massive amounts of soy beans and corn to support animal agriculture in the United States. This is a boon for genetically engineered farming as yields of corn, cotton, and soybeans are said to have risen by 20 to 30 percent through the use of genetic engineering. Meanwhile, the use of toxic herbicides, such as glyphosate in Roundup, has increased fifteenfold since GMOs were first introduced. That's good for business if the bottom line is enhancing your bottom line. In March 2015, the World Health Organization determined that the herbicide glyphosate is "probably carcinogenic to humans." A more recent study found a 41 percent increase in non-Hodgkin's lymphoma in those with high exposure to glyphosate. Adding credence to this association, in a prospective cohort study of more than sixty-eight thousand French volunteers, those who primarily ate organic foods were less likely to develop non-Hodgkin's lymphoma and postmenopausal breast cancer compared to those who rarely or never ate organic foods.

Why I buy organic whenever possible

By definition, if a food is certified organic it is not genetically modified and was not sprayed by glyphosate. I don't think this is the only reason to buy organic produce, however. I view it as an investment in my health, our family's health, and the health of our planet. The chemicals being used in modern agriculture aren't affecting only us; they're affecting the health of our soil. If you don't have healthy soil, you can't have nutritious food. Human health starts in the dirt. We need to protect this precious commodity. When you spend your money, you are placing your vote in a way. You are empowering an industry. I, for one, choose to empower our organic farmers and regenerative agriculture. They are healers just as our doctors are. Only with them can we enrich our soil, increase biodiversity, and heal ecosystems large (our planet) and small (your gut). Let's rally behind them and give them the support they deserve.

Let's take a step back for a moment and consider our modern life in the broader context of human evolution. Since the very first human, the microbes have been a part of our story. Every single human life has been a buddy tale about our relationship with our microbes. We rose and fell together. We coevolved. For most of the three million years we lived in a famished, violent world, exposed to the elements. Life was about survival, and most of us succumbed at a young age to infection, starvation, or bodily injury. We needed to live long enough to procreate and continue our species. If not, we'd go extinct. So our microbes helped us to develop an immune system to fight infection, clotting factors to stop bleeding, and efficient ways to harvest and store energy from our food. For example, the insulin resistance seen in type 2 diabetes is actually a protective mechanism to maintain fuel for the brain in times of starvation. As part of species preservation we evolved a taste for salt, sugar, and fat because in famine those promote survival. We became wired to crave those things.

Now consider the American college kid, lying on the couch all day playing video games, drinking soda, and having pizza delivered. The human experience is radically different in just the last hundred years. We've moved indoors, become sedentary, obsess over electronics, spray everything (including ourselves) with chemicals, and have a limitless food supply that exploits our taste for salt, sugar, and fat. And now the inflammation, clotting, and energy preservation that we needed to keep our species alive is the very thing causing cancer, cardiovascular disease, obesity, and diabetes. What once helped preserve our species has become our fatal flaw.*

And right now, as we speak, our microbes are evolving to adapt to the new environment. Given their central role in human health, we can either passively let them spin out of control with our destructive lifestyle, or we can embrace them as our "secret sauce" for longevity and healthy aging. My goal with this book is to help you shake off the detriments of a twenty-first-century life by engineering your microbiome for health and longevity. In order to do this, we need to pay attention to anything that disrupts the gut microbiota. Let's take a deeper dive into how the things we put into our mouth and swallow—medications and food—affect your gut health.

---

* This is referred to as "antagonistic pleiotropy," which means that a trait that can be helpful in certain circumstances proves to actually be harmful in other circumstances.

Modern health care, drugs, and your microbiota

It comes as no surprise that antibiotics absolutely decimate the gut microbiota. Just five days of ciprofloxacin wipes out about a third of gut bacteria and your gut microbiota are never quite the same. Most species recover within four weeks, but some are still absent after six months. In the case of clarithromycin and metronidazole, the effects are still evident four years after treatment. And just four days of three broad-spectrum antibiotics can permanently destroy nine beneficial species of bacteria. The result of all these antibiotics is a "new normal" microbiome with more antibiotic-resistant microbes that leaves us vulnerable to infection, allergic conditions, osteoporosis, and obesity. I'm sure you recall all the problems we had with antibiotics and *C. diff* infection up until we started using fecal transplant. Pretty disturbing stuff when you consider that there are 269 million antibiotic prescriptions in the United States each year and a recent study suggested that 23 percent of antibiotic prescriptions are flat-out inappropriate while another 36 percent were questionable.

Antibiotics aren't the only medicines causing trouble. In one study, 24 percent of tested drugs altered gut bacteria. For example, proton pump inhibitors increase the risk of small intestine bacterial overgrowth and *C. diff*. Nonsteroidal anti-inflammatory drugs (NSAIDs) like ibuprofen and naproxen alter the gut microbiota, destroy the intestinal lining to create ulcers, and predispose to inflammatory bowel disease and microscopic colitis. Oral contraceptives have been associated with the development of both Crohn's disease and ulcerative colitis. Frankly, these are just the tip of the iceberg. There are so many other medicines that I have concerns about, but the studies haven't been done yet.

The SAD diet is literally killing your gut

While medications are huge, let's not ignore the most important change over the last hundred years—our diet.

According to U.S. Department of Agriculture estimates, 32 percent of our calories come from animal foods, 57 percent from processed plant foods, and only 11 percent from whole grains, beans, fruits, vegetables, and nuts. The average American eats twenty-three pounds of pizza, twenty-four pounds of artificial sweeteners, twenty-nine pounds of french fries, and thirty-one pounds of cheese per year. The United States also has the highest meat consumption in the world—about 220 pounds of meat per person per year. We eat meat thirty-two times for every single time a person in India sits down to have it in their meal. Yet there are fad diets out there trying to convince you to double down on this trend. That it's not enough; we need more.

The Standard American Diet (SAD) stands in stark contrast to the people who live in the Blue Zones as described by Dan Buettner. These are the regions of the world where people are living much longer compared to the rest of us. There are five Blue Zones: Okinawa, Japan; Sardinia, Italy; Nicoya, Costa Rica; Icaria, Greece; and . . . *drumroll* . . . Loma Linda, California.

Wait, what? Cali? Yes, right here in our own country lives a group of people who use the same health care and the same food systems and they live ten years longer than most Americans on average. They are also ten times more likely to live to a hundred! Who are these mystery people? They are the Seventh-day Adventists, whose theology teaches them that they will come back to re-inhabit their bodies and therefore they emphasize health and self-care. They have proven that it's entirely possible to be a healthy American.

So here are these five geographic regions scattered around the world, completely culturally distinct, yet there are common themes in the food that they eat. All five are at least 90 percent plant-based. There's an emphasis on seasonal fruits and vegetables, legumes, whole grains, and nuts. Cow's milk is not a part of their diet, and meat is consumed sparingly, using it as a celebratory food, a small side, or a way to flavor dishes. In contrast, the Standard American Diet relies heavily on processed food, meat, and dairy pounded on our poor gut microbes three times a day with snacks and desserts to boot. What's it doing to us? Let's break down the science behind the elements:

Sugars and highly refined carbohydrates

The average American crushes 152 pounds of sugar *and* 120 pounds of grains per year, most of which are highly refined to strip away the fiber, causing them to be rapidly absorbed in the small intestine rather than slowly digested. Think white bread/rice/pasta and sugary cereals. These are not healthy carbohydrates! The result is a dramatic loss of gut microbial diversity and the rise of inflammatory bacteria that love simple carbohydrates. And then we wonder where our sugar cravings come from.

Salt

Processed foods are loaded to the gills with salt. The average American consumes nearly three pounds of salt per year. Three pounds! We only need a few ounces. Anything more has consequences, including in the gut microbiome, where it drives autoimmunity by inducing helper T cells, which can contribute to hypertension.

Chemical preservatives, additives, and colorants

Does it come as a surprise that the ten thousand food additives in our food supply may be destroying our microbiota? Numerous food additives have already been shown to damage the gut microbiota, while more than 99 percent of them haven't been studied. For example, two commonly used emulsifiers—carboxymethylcellulose and polysorbate 80—reduce microbial diversity, induce inflammation, and promote obesity and colitis in mice. Titanium dioxide (TiO) nanoparticles, found in more than nine hundred food products, worsen intestinal inflammation.

Additives such as these were snuck into our diet through the "Generally Recognized As Safe" loophole. They were GRASed into our diet. Yes, GRAS needs to be used as a verb because that's the only way to adequately describe the careless acceptance of chemicals into our food supply by our regulatory agencies.

Some would argue that if these chemicals are consumed in limited doses they are safe based on animal model studies. I strongly disagree. To GRAS is to assume safety until proven otherwise. That's a huge assumption given that animal models often don't translate to humans. We have no human studies for most of these ten thousand additives, and we definitely don't have long-term studies. Anyone who would claim confidence that these additives truly are safe for long-term human consumption would be doing so without human research to say so. There are ten thousand chances for us to be wrong in our assumption of safety, and it only takes us being wrong once to cause harm. Rather than GRASing things into our food supply and hoping for the best, I believe it best to be skeptical until actually proven otherwise.

Artificial sweeteners

"These artificial sweeteners are awesome! All the flavor, no calories!"
—Dr. B, 2013
"Keep that crap away from me!"—Dr. B, today

How about artificial sweeteners, ubiquitous in diet soda beverages and loads of other places? When they came to market we thought, "Zero calories, that *has* to be better than sugar, right?" It's intuitive! Turns out they're actually worse because they induce changes in the microbiome that promote inflammation, insulin resistance, and liver injury. You will actually be *less* tolerant of sugar by using artificial sweeteners.

And then there's the downright scary stuff . . . Remember from Chapter 1 the explosion of *Clostridioides difficile* that's occurred in the last twenty years? *C. diff* infection was fairly rare and only seen in hospitalized patients on antibiotics in the early 2000s. Just ten years later we're seeing five hundred thousand infections per year and thirty thousand deaths including in college kids who have never stepped foot in a hospital or had recent antibiotic use. Our antibiotics stopped working so we desperately reach for human feces, used as medicine, to save our butts. Literally. There has to be an explanation, right? Turns out that a dietary additive that you've probably never heard of called trehalose was GRASed into the American, European, and Canadian food supply in 2000, 2001, and 2005, respectively. Trehalose is a sweetener that the food industry loves because it improves the stability and texture of foods. It's used in pasta, ice cream, even beef. You can buy it by the kilogram on Amazon and throw it in your coffee. But a 2018 publication in *Nature* showed that: 1) trehalose promotes the growth of nasty, virulent strains of *C. diff* infection in an animal model; and 2) the timing of implementation of trehalose into our food supply coincides with the emergence of the *C. diff* epidemic with these exact strains worldwide. It took eighteen years for us to identify the problem. So has trehalose been taken off the market due to safety concerns? Unfortunately, no. "All you've shown is an association, without proof of harm in humans." See how that works? It will be very difficult to roll back the ten thousand food additives we've GRASed into existence.

Closing the book on processed foods

The thing about processed foods is that you're starting with something that's healthy in its natural state, and you are modifying it. As you progressively change that food, it becomes less and less nutritionally valuable. At some point, the food that started healthy becomes poison.

If you go back one hundred years, this simply wasn't a part of our diet. Take a moment to think about that: the sheer volume of man-made chemicals we're putting into our bodies, and the unrealistic expectation that our microbiota will be able to process and eliminate them without any damage. It's a shock that we don't drop dead from this stuff and a total testament to the adaptability of our microbiome, even if this is likely contributing to mass bacterial extinction.

It comes as no surprise that every 10 percent increase in consumption of ultra-processed foods is associated with *more* than a 10 percent increased risk of developing cancer and a 14 percent risk of early death. So what happens when you hit American levels of consumption—50 or 60 percent?

I don't think that every food additive is harmful in the long term, but we don't know and likely will never know. There's only one foolproof way to protect yourself from the potential poisons in our diet—get rid of them!

Unhealthy fats

Not all fats are unhealthy, but most of the fat in the American diet is of the unhealthy variety unfortunately. Study after study in an animal model has shown that a high-fat diet causes an unhealthy balance in the microbiota, impairs intestinal barrier function, and leads to the release of bacterial endotoxin. As you recall from Chapter 1, this is the model of dysbiosis, and bacterial endotoxin has been linked to autoimmunity, obesity, coronary artery disease, congestive heart failure, type 2 diabetes, Alzheimer's, alcoholic hepatitis, nonalcoholic fatty liver, osteoarthritis, and even "low T" in men.

Do the animal model findings translate to humans? Yes. A recent study in humans held dietary fiber constant and varied the amount of fat in the diet—20, 30, or 40 percent of calories. After six months they saw the microbiome shift to a progressively more inflammatory profile when fat was higher, confirmed with higher systemic inflammation. More fat, more problems.

So which fats are good and which are bad? The above study was done with vegetable oil, which can often be partially hydrogenated and high in trans fats. Other sources of trans fats are baked goods, chips, fried food, canned biscuits, nondairy creamer, and margarine. There is universal agreement that trans fats are unhealthy. Check the label for trans fats and don't buy it!

On the flip side, there is universal agreement that monounsaturated fats (MUFA) and omega-3 polyunsaturated fats (PUFA) found predominantly in plant foods are healthy! We see this validated in microbiome studies that show oleic acid—a monounsaturated fat found in olive oil—and omega-3 PUFAs promote the growth of beneficial microbes, correct dysbiosis, and reduce bacterial endotoxin release. They even enhance microbial diversity. These fats actually protect the microbiome.

And then there's saturated fat, predominantly found in animal foods as well as in tropical oils like coconut oil and palm oil. Cardiologists are screaming and shouting that it causes obesity, heart disease, and diabetes. Low-carb dieters disagree, and *Time* magazine says "Butter is back." But what does the microbiome say? The results in the microbiome have been consistent. Saturated fat encourages the growth of inflammatory microbes like *Bilophila wadsworthia*, alters intestinal permeability, and leads to the release of bacteria endotoxin. Translation: saturated fat causes dysbiosis. It even disrupts our normal biological rhythm in a way that promotes obesity. If you care about the health of your microbiome, then "Butter is not back" and we should probably rethink this ghee- and coconut-oil-in-the coffee fad.

Animal protein

"So where do you get your protein from?" That's the question that patients always ask when I discuss a plant-based diet with them. I get it. We've been taught that protein is the be-all and end-all of nutrition. Our obsession with protein fuels the heaviest meat consumption on the entire planet. But what's interesting is that "where you get your protein from" is incredibly important to gut health.

The source of the protein, whether from plants or animals, can have very different effects on the microbiome. For example, plant protein increases the growth of anti-inflammatory species like *Bifidobacterium* and *Lactobacillus* while suppressing the destructive ones like *Bacteroides fragilis* and *Clostridium perfringens*. The result is correction of leaky gut.

On the flip side, diets high in animal protein have consistently been associated with increased growth of inflammatory microbes like *Bilophila wadsworthia*, *Alistipes*, and *Bacteroides*. These bacteria produce toxins like amines, sulfides, and secondary bile salts. Amines cause food sensitivity at baseline, and then when you char meat it turns them into carcinogenic heterocyclic amines. Hydrogen sulfide has been associated with ulcerative colitis. Secondary bile salts have been associated with cancer of the colon, esophagus, stomach, small intestine, liver, pancreas, and biliary tract. No surprise, this consumption of animal protein results in increased intestinal permeability and inflammation.

And then there's the association between animal protein and TMAO, which has redefined our understanding of America's number one killer—cardiovascular disease. When people ingest L-carnitine (abundant in red meat and some energy drinks and supplements) or certain choline (found in red meat, liver, egg yolk, and dairy products), the gut bacteria produce trimethylamine N-oxide, or TMAO. Increased TMAO means increased risk of heart disease, stroke, Alzheimer's, type 2 diabetes, chronic kidney disease, peripheral artery disease, congestive heart failure, and atrial fibrillation—to name a few. Unhealthy food feeds unhealthy microbes that produce unhealthy compounds. It's a vicious cycle that's only broken by replacing unhealthy food with healthy food.

The good news is that a plant-based diet promotes a gut microbiota that just doesn't know how to make TMAO. Studies show that about four weeks after giving up red meat, people's TMAO levels drop dramatically. This explains why in *The Lifestyle Heart Trial,* Dr. Dean Ornish showed that through a low-fat vegetarian diet, smoking cessation, stress management, and moderate exercise, patients actually *reversed* coronary artery disease. Meanwhile the control group got worse and worse.

What's interesting is that increased animal protein can produce weight loss in the short term but causes a shift in the microbiome that's bad for our gut health in the long term. I suppose now would be a good time to have a little chat about the fad diets that offer weight loss in exchange for heavy meat consumption . . .

Fad Diets

Let me make this clear . . . I don't look down on people who do fad diets. In fact, I applaud them for having the courage to change their diet in an effort to be healthier. But the million-dollar question is, "Are these diets good for your microbes?"

Let's start with the Paleo diet, our most popular and most often recommended dietary approach today. The idea is that we should eat the way our ancestors ate because modern agriculture is at odds with our ancestral biology. That means meat, eggs, vegetables, fruit, nuts, and roots are on the menu while dairy, sugars, grains, legumes, processed oils, salt, alcohol, and coffee are not. Some of this I love; some of this I don't.

But who cares what I think? Let's look at the science. In a recent study, consumption of a long-term Paleolithic diet was associated with dramatically higher TMAO levels, reduced *Roseburia* (protects against inflammatory bowel disease), reduced *Bifidobacterium* (protects against irritable bowel and obesity), and increased *Hungatella* (produces TMAO). In other words, the Paleo diet shifted the microbiome away from health and toward disease. Even though all of the groups in the study ate a similar amount of meat, they saw dramatic differences in the amount of TMAO produced, with the highest level being in those who were most strict in following the Paleo diet. Elimination of whole grains was the main factor responsible for increased *Hungatella* and TMAO levels, demonstrating that categorical eliminations can have unintended, potentially serious consequences.

Anyone want to guess what an even more restrictive Keto/Carnivore diet does to the microbiome? In a groundbreaking study by Drs. Lawrence David and Peter Turnbaugh, a group of people cycled between a completely "plant-based diet," which was rich in grains, legumes, fruits, and vegetables, and an "animal-based diet," which was composed of meats, eggs, and cheeses. This "animal-based diet" could also be called the "Keto diet"—extremely low carb, very high fat. It could also be called the "Carnivore diet"—100 percent animal products, no plants.

So what happened? There were dramatic changes of the study's participants in the microbiome in less than twenty-four hours. It didn't take long. The animal-based diet saw the disturbing emergence of inflammatory bacteria like *Bilophila wadsworthia*, *Alistipes putredinis*, and *Bacteroides*. This was expected with high levels of saturated fat and animal protein. Remember, these are the bacteria that produce toxins like amines, sulfides, and secondary bile salts. Meanwhile, there was starvation and recession of the healing microbes like *Roseburia*, *Eubacterium rectale*, and *Faecalibacterium prausnitzii*. Similar to the Paleo diet, this is a shift away from health and toward disease. Perhaps the most disturbing part is the rapid emergence of *Bilophila wadsworthia*, known to produce hydrogen sulfide, which promotes inflammatory bowel disease. It's alarming to consider that in less than five days the foundation is being laid for the development of Crohn's disease or ulcerative colitis with this diet.

But these low-carb, high-fat diets are helping people to lose weight, right? Folks, we have to learn that you can lose weight, look great on the outside, and be absolutely rotting on the inside. It's short-term gain and long-term pain. Do you know the average life expectancy of a professional body builder? It's just forty-seven years. Weight loss doesn't always translate into better health.

To view the 55+ scientific references cited in this chapter, please visit me online at www.theplantfedgut.com/research/.

3

The Fiber Solution: Short-Chain Fatty Acids and Postbiotics for the Win

Our guts are STARVING to be Fiber Fueled

So what can we do to restore order and bring out the best in our 'biota? Where do we begin if we want to heal our guts to reverse or prevent illness? Is it probiotics? Bone broth?

Well, if you were sitting across from me in my office, I'd be going straight for my secret weapon—fiber. I know what you're thinking. "Fiber? Really? Fiber is, like, the most boring thing on the entire planet, Dr. B," or "You mean that gross white powder my grandma mixes into a glass of water every morning so she can poop?"

And to that I'd say: Fair enough. Fiber has gotten a bad rap, and those tasteless fiber supplements are only partly to blame. It's also the fact that until very recently we had absolutely no idea just how amazing fiber is for your gut microbiota. You most likely have preconceived notions about it that make it hard for me to make fiber cool or sexy. For a while now, the diet conversation has been all about protein and, more recently, fat. Nobody has been talking about boring old fiber. I'm here to tell you that fiber is the first, and potentially the most powerful, solution to restoring health to your gut microbiota, and from there your overall health.

But for this to work I need you to unlearn what you think you already know. I'm not talking about fiber as you know it. It's time for a reboot. A renaissance. A rebranding. It's time to stop thinking about fiber as being vanilla and boring and get to know it in a whole new light. Fiber is so much more than you once thought it was. Yes, fiber is the real deal, folks. If by the end of this chapter you want to intentionally mispronounce it as "FIRE," I don't blame you. I'm going to resist that urge for this book, but if we ever meet in person I hope you'll shake my hand and tell me the secret code, "Fiber is FIRE."

Did you know that 97 percent of us consume an excess of protein, yet we still constantly ask, "Where am I going to get my protein from?" We live in a country with a pathologic protein obsession. Meanwhile, we are figuratively and literally starving for fiber. "Starving?" you say. "In this country? Where nearly three in four are overweight?" Absolutely. Your gut is completely FIBER STARVED. Imagine your gut as a dried-out, postapocalyptic wasteland, with a lone tumbleweed rolling through. That solitary tumbleweed represents your fiber! Less than 3 percent of Americans get even the recommended *minimum* daily intake. That means 97 percent of Americans are not receiving the *minimal* daily recommended amount of fiber, let alone what I would characterize as optimal. Of all of the essential nutrients, this may be our greatest, most prevalent deficiency. Yet, we're not talking about it and no one seems to be concerned. Enough with the protein obsession; it's time we turn our attention to the vital question: "Where am I going to get my fiber from?"

Fiber, the phoenix: Let's burn it down and watch it come back stronger!

Okay, taking it from the top: What is fiber? In nature, fiber is a part of the plant cellular structure. Plants have a total monopoly on this nutrient. So if you want it, there's only one way to naturally get it: from plants!

From a nutritional perspective, fiber is a carb—it's what we would refer to as a complex carbohydrate. If you take multiple sugar molecules and link them together, you'd get fiber. That doesn't mean it behaves like sugar by any means. It doesn't. Digestion of refined sugar starts in the mouth and in about twenty minutes it's already been absorbed in the small intestine. Meanwhile, fiber remains unblemished as it passes through your mouth, stomach, and even fifteen to twenty feet of small intestine so that by the time it reaches your colon, it's the same molecule that went in your mouth.

Two of the biggest myths about fiber are that all fiber is the same and that it does nothing more than go in one end and shoot out the other like a torpedo. Let's dig deeper.

Have you turned into a carbophobic?

If just seeing the word "carb" gets your heart racing and your face flushing, then it's happened. But don't worry; it's not your fault. There's been so much negative press for carbs. They're not very "in" and they haven't been for quite some time. You've been taught that carbs are bad for you; they spike your blood sugar, increase your food cravings, and you need to avoid them if you want to lose weight. Is it true? Sometimes. But not in whole food form.

Yes, refined, processed carbs like table sugar or high-fructose corn syrup, white bread or white flour will spike your blood sugar, leading to a vicious cycle of food addiction, weight gain, and constant hunger. That's because they've been stripped of their fiber. As you're about to learn, fiber is directly responsible for balancing our blood sugar and triggering our satiety hormones so that we know when to say, "That's enough, thank you."

Complex, unrefined carbs found in whole plant foods are chock-full of fiber, vitamins, and minerals. In contrast to that vicious cycle above, complex carbs actually lower blood sugar—even prevent diabetes—and decrease weight and body mass. The point is that we shouldn't make assumptions about our food based upon macro- or micronutrients. We need to look at whole foods. The fear surrounding carbs is appropriately placed with the refined carbs in processed foods, but completely misplaced with the unrefined carbs found in whole plant foods. Seriously, fruit is *actually* the low-hanging fruit!

Myth #1: All fiber is the same, and all you have to do is count grams.

You've been taught that all fiber is created equal—that whether it's in your breakfast cereal, the milky powder your grandma drinks, or in a granola bar, all forms of fiber are interchangeable. All you need to do is count the number of grams and you're good to go. What you've been told is dead wrong.

The source of the fiber you eat is critically important. The fiber in your cereal or breakfast biscuit is not the same as the fiber in your quinoa. This is conceptually similar to how the source of our fats and our protein determines the impact on our microbiome. It's an over-simplification to reduce fiber to a number of grams and pretend that all grams are created equal. As you're going to learn in Chapter 4, I have a much better way to source your fiber.

We've been taught to count grams of fiber for two reasons. One, it's easy, and we like easy. And two, we have no clue how many types of fiber actually exist in nature. It's incredibly difficult to analyze the chemical structure of dietary fiber, and there are four hundred thousand plants on our planet, three hundred thousand of them being edible. So there must be hundreds of thousands—if not millions—of types of fiber in nature. But we haven't gotten around to figuring them all out yet.

Given the complexities in analyzing dietary fiber, we've simplified it by saying there are two basic forms of dietary fiber: soluble and insoluble. You can tell which is which by submerging the fiber in water. If it dissolves, it's soluble. If it doesn't, it's insoluble. While I will occasionally make references to the difference between soluble and insoluble fiber, just know that in both cases we are talking about huge categories of fiber and that most plants contain some mix of both.

Myth #2: That fiber just passes through us.

If you do a quick Google search on fiber, you'll find the general health benefits of fiber: It contributes to fantastic bowel movements by correcting diarrhea and constipation and increasing the weight and size of your bowel movement, lowers cholesterol, and controls blood sugar. These are all great things, and we should be celebrating these health benefits of fiber, for sure! But at the same time we have been doing the undersell of the century here, folks.

We've all been taught that fiber pretty much goes in the mouth and out your . . . well, you know, and along the way it sweeps some stuff out. And while there may be some truth to these statements, we're being excessively simple about an incredibly complicated nutrient. So let's take a closer look.

We humans lack the ability to process fiber by ourselves. Sure, we've got some enzymes called glycoside hydrolases that help us break down complex carbs, but we only have seventeen of them—just seventeen!—and none of them are designed for breaking down the larger molecules like fiber. In other words, we big strong humans are literally incapable of processing fiber on our own.

Now, if we lived encapsulated in a sterile bubble free from bacteria, we would never know the true power of fiber. But we get by with a little help from our friends. Because guess where you can find lots and lots of fiber and complex carbohydrate-processing enzymes? Yes, in our gut microbiota. Compared to the shockingly inadequate seventeen that belong to us, our gut microbiota may contain upward of sixty thousand of these helpful enzymes.

The fact that our microbiomes contain this insane number of digestive enzymes makes sense when you remember that there are three hundred thousand edible plants and potentially millions of types of fiber in our diet. By outsourcing fiber digestion to our microbes, we are taking advantage of their adaptability. Every single plant, every single type of fiber requires a unique team of microbes working in concert to get the job done. It's demanding work, but what follows is magic. The breakdown of fiber by gut bacteria unleashes what I believe is the most healing nutrient in all of nature: (*Drumroll, please!*) short-chain fatty acids (SCFAs).

Short-chain fatty acids (SCFAs) to the rescue

We've learned about our "good bacteria." But how do these powerful microbes actually do their incredible work? Good bacteria have the ability to transform certain types of fiber into electric, organic power manna—they're called SCFAs.

There are three main types of SCFAs: acetate, propionate, and butyrate. These are literally as they are described: short-chain, meaning made up of two, three, or four carbon atoms connected together in acetate, propionate, and butyrate chemical compounds, respectively. The three SCFAs work in the body as a complementary group. In the interest of understanding them better we generally study them in isolation, but always keep in mind that there are studies and then there's real life. In real life, these molecules are meant to work together, in the proper balance, for the good of your health.

Each type of fiber we consume produces a different mix of these

SCFAs when processed by good bacteria. But don't worry about trying to get specific ones for specific problems—the key here, which you'll learn all about in Chapter 4, is to consume a diverse mix of fibers, meaning a diverse mix of plants, to get the benefits of *all of them*.

The different "-biotics" for gut health: pre, pro, and post

Before we go any further into the science of SCFAs I want to explain something. I'm sure you've heard of probiotics; we've all seen those yogurt commercials. Probiotics are all the rage and have been for some time. But have you ever heard of prebiotics or postbiotics? In short, probiotics are living bacteria that have been demonstrated to have beneficial qualities to us humans. Prebiotics induce the growth or beneficial qualities of the probiotics. They're essentially food for the good bugs. Postbiotics are the healthy compounds produced by bacterial metabolism.

In other words:

Prebiotics = Food for healthy gut microbes
Probiotics = Microbes with beneficial qualities
Postbiotics = Compounds produced by gut microbes

Taken a step further . . .
Prebiotics + Probiotics = Postbiotics

The word "prebiotic" literally did not exist until 1995, but it is increasingly becoming a part of the American vernacular. It is defined as "a substrate that is selectively utilized by host microorganisms conferring a health benefit." In other words, prebiotics (the substrate) are utilized by the microorganisms (probiotics) to confer a health benefit by producing postbiotics. Which is just the nerdy way of saying my formula: prebiotics + probiotics = postbiotics.

Not all fiber is prebiotic. Most soluble fiber is prebiotic, while most insoluble fiber is not. We often call insoluble fiber roughage. The roughage is the part that's untouched by our digestion or our microbes, and therefore launches out the bottom like a torpedo.

Fiber isn't the only prebiotic though! Resistant starch, found in foods like oats, rice, potatoes, and legumes, is technically not fiber but it behaves in a very similar way to soluble fiber. It passes through the small intestine unblemished and is fermented by our colon microbes. A mother's breast milk also contains something called human milk oligosaccharides, or HMOs, that function like soluble fiber and feed the baby's developing gut microbiota. So if we want postbiotic SCFAs, we should get prebiotic soluble fiber and resistant starch in our diet and we should breastfeed our young ones.

All roads point to SCFAs for human health. They are the dominant driver of gut health and they have benefits throughout the body.

Going beyond fiber for next-level prebiotics

While fiber is a strong and reliable source for prebiotics, healthy prebiotics exist in other plant compounds as well. The healing properties of numerous plants—including cocoa, green and black tea, pomegranate, apples, and blueberries—are at least partially attributable to phytochemical polyphenols, which are antioxidant compounds. Ninety to 95 percent of polyphenols make their way down to the colon, where they're magically transformed by our microbes and activated to their health-promoting form. Similarly, omega-3 polyunsaturated fatty acids found in walnuts have been shown to be prebiotic. Yay, healthy fats! So while polyphenols and omega-3's don't produce short-chain fatty acids like fiber, they do have an effect on our gut microbes and cause the release of health-promoting compounds, also known as postbiotics.

Nutritional karma and the power of positive momentum

Now let's come back to SCFAs, your good gut bacteria, and fiber. Healthy bacteria can't survive without fiber. In fact, studies have shown that fiber consumption increases the growth of healthy bacteria species such as *Lactobacilli, Bifidobacteria,* and *Prevotella.* Eating fiber also increases the diversity of species within the gut. These beneficial effects are what qualify it as a prebiotic. The prebiotic effects of fiber feed and nourish the healthy microbes in our gut. Your gut bacteria goes from slumped over and worn out to energized, steadfast, and powerful.

Those reinvigorated microbes release SCFAs from fiber to heal the colon. First, the short-chain fatty acids do as their name suggests and make the colon more acidic. This change prevents the growth of inflammatory, pathogenic bacteria—the bad guys. Next, SCFAs take it a step further and directly suppress dangerous strains like *E. coli* and *Salmonella.* In Chapter 1 we learned that dysbiosis is characterized by a loss of balance between the healthy microbes and the inflammatory ones. By suppressing inflammatory microbes, SCFAs are helping to restore that balance.

Now we're building momentum toward a healthier gut. Fiber is feeding the healthy microbes, and they're multiplying. As they increase in number, they're producing more and more SCFAs for us even though you're consuming the same amount of fiber. You have trained your gut to produce SCFAs, and it's become increasingly efficient at doing that. These SCFAs are suppressing the inflammatory microbes, giving the healthy microbes an even more decisive advantage over the inflammatory ones. This is a form of positive health momentum, and it starts building on itself as we get more and more healthy microbes producing more and more SCFAs. But keep in mind, the linchpin here is fiber. Everything I've described is contingent on fueling your gut microbes with prebiotic fiber.

As you can see, regular consumption of fiber trains your gut microbiome not only to process fiber, but to actually get even more beneficial postbiotics out of it! In exercise we call it muscle memory. In life we call it practice. Either way, our microbes are no different. If you regularly expose them to fiber in your diet, they will adapt to that regular exposure and get really, really good at extracting SCFAs for you. With that comes a myriad of benefits that I'm just starting to tell you about.

But here's the problem—the flip side is also true: a diet lacking in fiber will drain your gut of its fiber-extracting capabilities and make it less capable of getting postbiotics from your food. When you don't practice, you lose your skill, right? Just two weeks on a low-fiber diet causes an altered gut microbiota that starts to literally eat away at the intestinal lining, causing breakdown of the protective barrier and susceptibility to disease. Not good. And remember how I said that 97 percent of us aren't even getting minimal fiber? And that six of the top ten causes of death in the United States are caused by nutrition? And that most of those are linked with dysbiosis of the gut? You're starting to get the FIRE for fiber burning a little now, aren't you?

This is a really key point that I want to get across. You can call it nutritional karma—"do good and you will receive good." Or you could say that you're not what you eat but what your gut microbiota eats. The point is that your food choices leave an imprint in your microbiome and those choices will either train your gut bacteria to take care of and protect you or empower evildoers to hurt you. Your choice.

What else can SCFAs do? Well, they also fix up your colonocytes, which are the cells lining your colon. Maybe you've been led to believe that fiber provides no energy since it's not absorbed? Believe it or not, 10 percent of our daily caloric requirements are met with fiber-derived SCFAs as the energy source. In fact, the main source of energy for our colonocytes are SCFAs, providing up to 70 percent of their energy. Specifically, the colonocytes seem to love chowing down on the SCFA butyrate, so most of the butyrate is taken up by the gut lining where it contributes to a healthy colon. Like taking a beautiful historic home that's been run haggard and restoring it to its original glory, butyrate fixes up the lining of the gut.

"Doc, how do I fix leaky gut?" Here is your solution.

Back in Chapter 1 we talked about dysbiosis, which is when damage to the gut microbiota causes increased intestinal permeability, which leads to release of noxious bacterial endotoxin. Remember that the gut wall is meant to act like a physical barrier exerting control over what stuff gets access to your blood. After all, it's in the gut that your body is most exposed to the outside world. This blood–gut barrier is meant for protection, but holes can occur in the wall allowing bacteria, antigens, and toxic substances like bacterial endotoxin to get past the intestinal wall, activating the immune system. This increased intestinal permeability, which some refer to as "leaky gut," happens when tight junction proteins that are meant to keep cells connected to one another end up being broken, thereby creating gaps between the cells. Good news: SCFA butyrate actually *repairs* leaky gut by increasing the expression of tight junction proteins and has been shown to actually decrease endotoxin release.

And while we're on the topic, inflammation caused by increased intestinal permeability affects the function of the intestinal lining, including its nerves and muscles. This leads to diarrhea or constipation, bloating, and abdominal pain. Unfortunately, even just transient inflammation of the gut and intestinal hyperpermeability can cause sensitization and altered motility that persists long after resolution of the inflammation. You may recall from Chapter 1 that the hallmarks of irritable bowel syndrome are altered gut motility and increased visceral hypersensitivity. SCFA butyrate has been shown to increase colonic motility and decrease visceral hypersensitivity. So if you suffer from IBS, then you want this.

Let's take a step back for a moment here, folks. What I'm telling you is that SCFAs are a *vital nutrient* for intestinal health. They are the dominant energy source for your colon, support a healthy gut microbiota, repair leaky gut, reduce release of bacterial endotoxin, promote intestinal motility, and decrease visceral hypersensitivity. Read that sentence again: Let it sink in. I just described the cure for dysbiosis. I believe that dysbiosis is at the root of most modern disease. SCFAs can correct dysbiosis, and that's only the beginning of the health benefits they offer.

If correcting dysbiosis, supporting a healthy gut microbiota, repairing your colon, and reversing leaky gut weren't enough, this superhero energy fans out throughout the body and works its healing magic. Let's take a look at some of the most impressive capabilities of SCFAs beyond the gut.

Immune system and inflammation

Just beyond the wall of your intestine sits 70 percent of your immune system. This is your little army. When infection or even cancerous cells arise, it is the responsibility of your immune system to clear it out. Sounds simple, but it's not. How do you separate friend from foe when there are thirty-nine trillion microbes in the gut, thirty trillion human cells in the body, and your "host" is scarfing down three pounds of food per day, most of which is some deviant form of real food? That's a ton of responsibility. The slightest bit of confusion by the immune system leads to failure. Overreact and you get allergic or autoimmune issues. Underreact and you get infections or even cancer. So how do we get it juuuusssssttttttt right?

Well, SCFAs are the way that our gut microbiome connects to our immune system. It's how they communicate with each other. SCFAs act as a crisis negotiator, getting the immune system to cool off if it's too hot.

Dysbiosis and the release of bacterial endotoxin promote inflammation, which is a good thing when you have an infection or injury but isn't good when it's constant and unneeded. It's unrelenting low-grade stress on the body, including the immune system. Thankfully, SCFAs address both dysbiosis and bacterial endotoxin release, which makes them a great first step toward regulating the root cause of all inflammatory conditions.

Beyond that, SCFAs have been shown to inhibit three of the most powerful inflammatory signals in the body: NF-κB, IFN-γ, and TNF-α. I've heard people say that "your genes load the gun and your lifestyle pulls the trigger." If that's the case, then SCFAs disarm the gun and take it out of your hand. SCFAs make immune cells more tolerant to gut bacteria and reduce gut inflammatory markers. Believe it or not, they even make immune cells more tolerant to your food, helping to prevent food allergy and sensitivity. SCFAs can even communicate directly to an important part of our immune system called regulatory T cells, which you can think of as "suppressor" cells that cool off the immune system, encourage tolerance to your own cells, and prevent autoimmune disease. More on that in a bit.

We've seen more evidence of the power of fiber fueled SCFAs against inflammation in studying patients with Crohn's disease, a form of inflammatory bowel disease (IBD). In Crohn's, the immune system attacks the intestine, causing inflammation. It can affect any part of the digestive tract, from your lips to your backside. The inflammation in Crohn's can be so severe that it can actually erode through the wall of the intestine and cause abscesses or a connection between two parts that isn't supposed to exist, which we call a fistula. Suffice it to say that Crohn's is a horrible, debilitating condition that is becoming increasingly common in the Western world.

So let's take a look at how Crohn's disease develops and you'll see how SCFAs could make a difference. In people with Crohn's, we see decreased bacterial diversity, loss of butyrate-producing organisms, specifically *Faecalibacterium prausnitzii*, and an overgrowth of pathogenic bacteria, specifically *E. coli*. But this isn't just any *E. coli*. . . . No, no, no. This is an extra-nasty variety called adherent-invasive *E. coli*. Gives me the chills typing it, that's how nasty it is. Anyway, this *E. coli* behaves like a sociopath just broken out of prison, and immediately starts unleashing pro-inflammatory proteins like a flamethrower as it proliferates, further enhancing dysbiosis and the rise of more *E. coli*. This loss of balance in the gut, decrease in good bacteria, and increase in *E. coli* affects the tight junctions and leads to increased intestinal permeability. There is a strong association between depletion of *F. prausnitzii* and the immune system no longer being tolerant of the intestinal microbiota, meaning the immune system starts going haywire. Meanwhile, the absent intestinal barrier allows *E. coli* to invade the intestinal wall, which activates the immune system to attack the *E. coli*. And there you have it—inflammatory bowel disease.

As you can see, just like in life, when bad things happen in the body it's a series of events that lead to the problem. If we were functioning in the business world, we'd do a root cause analysis to figure out the source of the problem and address it. Could a *fiber-starved* gut be the root cause of Crohn's disease?

Well, yes: SCFAs are relevant in protection from Crohn's disease on a mechanistic level because they make immune cells more tolerant to gut bacteria, help suppress an overactive immune system, repair leaky gut, and create protective bacteria to keep the gut healthy. Additionally, in a recent study a semi-vegetarian high-fiber diet basically crushed an omnivorous diet in terms of keeping people with Crohn's disease free of disease activity and in remission. Those on a semi-vegetarian diet maintained a 92 percent remission rate compared to just 33 percent among omnivores in a prospective trial.

And in similar fashion, what if a high-fiber, plant-centered diet proved to be beneficial for other autoimmune, inflammatory conditions? Well, it does. In humans, a vegan diet has repeatedly been demonstrated to be beneficial for disease remission in rheumatoid arthritis. For example, in a randomized controlled trial 41 percent of patients on a vegan diet showed clinical improvement of their rheumatoid arthritis compared to just 4 percent on a "well-balanced" nonvegan diet.

So not only do SCFAs correct dysbiosis and heal leaky gut, but they also create a powerful link between the microbiome and immune system that serves to make the immune system work properly. Adequately fueled by SCFAs, the immune system does its job confidently and effectively. Without the SCFAs, the immune system becomes insecure, confused, paranoid, and weak. In other words, the immune system is dependent on gut microbes to support it with SCFAs. The gut microbes are dependent on you to offer fiber fuel that can be transformed into SCFAs. Again, these gut microbes aren't just passively along for the ride. They play an active, central role in our health.

Cancer

As we've learned, SCFAs correct dysbiosis, fix leaky gut, reverse bacterial endotoxemia, and optimize the immune system. Those effects create a good foundation for the prevention of cancer. We know from Chapter 1 that dysbiosis has been associated with several types of cancer: colorectal, gastric, esophageal, pancreatic, laryngeal, gallbladder, and even breast cancer. But is there anything special about SCFAs that can help us in the fight against cancer beyond just "healing the gut"?

Let's start with the basic premise that cancer development requires unchecked cell multiplication and growth. In order for this to happen, the DNA in the malignant cell needs to be able to copy itself before dividing into two cells. Histone deacetylases, or HDACs, are required to allow this process to occur. So if you could shut down the DNA copy process by blocking the HDACs, you'd effectively be pulling the emergency brake on the runaway cancer train.

Since the 1970s we've known that butyrate inhibits HDACs, altering gene expression in malignant cells and, as a result, inhibiting the root of cancer formation—unchecked proliferation. But when you have dangerous cells that you're dealing with, it's not enough to just slow down their growth. You need to stop them in their tracks, and the way this is done is by causing apoptosis, or programmed cell death. Sounds violent, but it's actually a normal part of cellular regulation and is by no means rare. Every day between fifty and seventy billion cells fall on the sword in altruistic fashion to protect the greater good of the whole organism. SCFAs help us in the fight against cancer by specifically eliminating cells that could turn into cancer.

Once again, studies on people who consume a high-fiber, plant-centered diet and reduce their cancer risk offer proof that these principles really translate to our real life. Let's go straight to the source and start with the most powerful, most well-respected study on the topic by Dr. Andrew Reynolds in *The Lancet*. He pulled information together from 243 prospective studies. This is a scale that is rarely seen in clinical research, yet at the same time he restricted his data to high-quality studies: prospective cohorts and interventional randomized trials. In the end, fiber found in whole foods was shown to protect against colorectal, breast, and esophageal cancer. Further, high dietary fiber in the study was still pretty low—between 25 and 29 grams per day. In the Western world, our fiber consumption is so poor that even the high-fiber consumers are below goal. Nonetheless, the results suggested that as you extend your dietary fiber intake higher, the protection against colorectal and breast cancer only gets greater.

Colon cancer is the number two cause of cancer death in the United States right now. Number two! And that's despite billions of dollars spent on our colon cancer screening program. Dietary fiber has been *repeatedly* shown to protect us from colon cancer. For example, in a prospective study of 1,575 people with nonmetastatic colorectal cancer, consuming more dietary fiber helped people live longer. For every 5 grams of increased fiber consumption, there was an 18 percent lower risk of death from colorectal cancer and 14 percent lower risk of death from any cause during follow-up.

And just to put the cherry on top, three major studies—a large 2017 meta-analysis, the prospective EPIC-Oxford study, and the Adventist Health Study—all reached the same conclusion when it comes to diet and cancer risk. A plant-centered, fiber fueled diet lowers your risk of developing cancer. Mic drop.

Heart Disease, Stroke, Diabetes, and Weight Loss

So SCFAs and fiber offer protection from cancer, the number two cause of death in the United States. How about heart disease and stroke—the number one and number five causes of death? In the same mega meta-analysis on dietary fiber published in *The Lancet*, Dr. Reynolds and his science squad also found dietary fiber consumption to be associated with lower body weight, reduced incidence of type 2 diabetes, lower total cholesterol, and lower systolic blood pressure. These just so happen to be the risk factors for coronary artery disease and stroke.

SCFAs affect multiple tissues in a concerted action to improve blood sugar regulation. They help protect against glucose intolerance, improve insulin response in the pancreas, and suppress fatty acids in the liver and peripheral tissues. This isn't exactly a revolutionary concept. There are studies dating back to the 1980s suggesting that soluble fiber is protective against type 2 diabetes. But modern studies, such as the recent *Science* article by Dr. Liping Zhao, dug more deeply and have shown us that following a high-fiber diet promotes the growth of SCFA-producing microbes that improve blood sugar regulation.

It's not just what you eat but the effect it has on your microbiota that determines your diabetes risk. There's something that was originally called the "lentil effect," but now we call it the "second meal effect," that illustrates this idea. If you give two people an amount of bread or lentils for lunch that have the same number of calories, you will of course see less of a sugar spike with the lentils. No surprise. But then these two people both have white bread for dinner, you'll *still* see less of a sugar spike in the person who had lentils for lunch. Same meal at dinner, but different effects based upon what you ate for lunch. We now understand that this happens because the bacteria that we empowered at lunch are working their SCFA magic to protect us at dinner. Score one for legumes, if you're keeping track.

SCFAs also lower cholesterol by having direct control over the critical enzyme in cholesterol formation and by increasing excretion of cholesterol in bile. Further, SCFAs directly activate a receptor in fat cells that decreases fatty acid uptake, and therefore suppresses fat accumulation.

Each of these mechanisms protects you from obesity. Additionally, SCFAs promote the release of satiety hormones that tell you when you've had enough. This is a wildly underrated benefit that we are sacrificing with our current highly processed, low-fiber diet. It allows you to feel nice and adequately full without crossing the line to where you need a pair of sweatpants, a three-hour nap, and an energy drink to get your day back on track. (Not that there's anything wrong with sweatpants!) When you are eating real food, nature works the way it's supposed to and you simply stop eating at the right time without counting calories and without overeating. As proof of concept, a randomized crossover study recently showed people experienced greater satiety and increased satiety hormones after eating a plant-based burger with tofu than after eating a pork and cheese burger, even though the two meals were matched for energy and macronutrients. Same number of calories, same macros, but better appetite control with the plants. Shocking, right?

Finally, patients with symptomatic coronary artery disease have been found to have depleted levels of butyrate-producing gut bacteria. In animal models SCFAs have been shown to protect against congestive heart failure and high blood pressure. More recently they've also been shown to prevent atherosclerosis by maintaining gut barrier function and limiting bacterial endotoxin release, which leads to less vascular inflammation. A recent study in humans with congestive heart failure found an absence of SCFA-producing microbes and an increase in TMAO-producing microbes. These patients had less butyrate and more TMAO coursing through their blood. And so we now understand at least in part why a plant-centered diet is good for the heart. SCFAs are the antithesis of TMAO.

Cognition

Like a Roman warrior throwing a spear, the superhero bacteria in our gut also unleash SCFAs all the way upstairs to the brain. What's interesting is that many molecules cannot travel to the brain due to a wall of protection called the blood–brain barrier. Most molecules are stopped there at the wall, like being stopped at the VIP line at the most exclusive club in New York City. (I wouldn't know what that's like because I'm a nerd and have never been, but I watched enough *Entourage* to at least be able to pretend.) So imagine that when the SCFAs show up, the velvet rope is withdrawn and they're given free access to the hottest club, our most precious organ, the brain.

On the other side of that velvet rope, SCFAs continue to work their magic. The same chemical that reverses dysbiosis, heals leaky gut, strengthens the gut microbiota, optimizes the immune system, and regulates appetite and metabolism also connects the gut microbiome to cerebral function. The effects are once again broad and powerful.

You know how many people with leaky gut also complain of brain fog? And how we also discussed above that SCFAs can activate tight junction proteins to repair increased permeability in the gut? Well, it appears that SCFAs work similar magic on the blood–brain barrier.

SCFA butyrate has demonstrated a profound effect on improving learning and memory. This has been demonstrated in models of

Alzheimer's, heavy metal toxicity, traumatic brain injury, and even neurologic infections (which sounds terrifying). I will tell you first-hand that the mental clarity that I've had since changing my diet has been life changing for me. Being totally real, there's no way I could've written this book before. I didn't have the stamina, focus, or neural plasticity.

Speaking of Alzheimer's, one of the hallmarks of Alzheimer's disease is the accumulation of amyloid plaques between nerve cells in the brain. Researchers are currently working on treatments for Alzheimer's to block the production of amyloid. Millions if not billions of dollars are being spent on this. While they continue that quest, I want you to know that laboratory studies suggest that SCFAs interfere with the formation of this exact same amyloid.

Laboratory studies also show that butyrate protects the brain in models of Parkinson's disease. This is quite interesting when you consider that human studies have found that patients with Parkinson's disease have lower levels of the bacteria that produce SCFAs and, as expected, lower levels of SCFAs in their stool. For what it's worth, Parkinson's disease patients almost all have digestive issues, with constipation being the most common among them.

Finally, children on a high-fiber diet demonstrate better cognitive control (multitasking, working memory, and maintaining focus) than children who eat a lower-fiber diet. So SCFAs may help ADHD. I'd far rather kids eat a salad than take Ritalin.

Bringing back fiber

Dr. Justin Sonnenburg showed that Westernization has led to a loss of gut microbial diversity in his study that compares the Hadza of Tanzania to Americans. The Hadza are one of the last remaining hunter-gatherer societies on the planet and provide insights into what our life and our microbiome may have looked like in primitive times. They consume 100 or more grams of fiber a day in their food, and during a year will include around six hundred plants in their diet. The average American gets a pathetic 15 grams of fiber per day and has fifty or fewer species of plants in their diet. The differences in the microbiota are profound. The Hadza have about 40 percent more diversity than the average American and about 30 percent more diversity than the average Brit.

Consider that African Americans have sixty-five times more colon cancer than rural Africans. Sixty-five times! One interesting study involved switching the diets of a group of African Americans and native Africans for two weeks. The Africans did a high-fat, low-fiber diet while the African Americans did a high-fiber, low-fat diet. Do you want to guess what happened?

When the native Africans began eating our American diet, they saw their SCFA butyrate levels decline and their TMAO levels increase. The reciprocal effect ended up being true for the African Americans. "Africanization" of the diet increased butyrate by 2.5-fold while "Westernization" cut butyrate quantities in half. Remember how secondary bile salts are known to cause colon cancer? A typical African diet reduced colonic secondary bile acids by 70 percent, while the Western diet increased them by 400 percent.

One last little mind-blowing nugget I want to leave you with: Dr. Sonnenburg also did a mouse study showing that the Western diet induced loss of microbial diversity that could be compounded over a series of generations. If your grandmother had twelve hundred species of microbes in her gut as a child, but by the time your mother was born she had nine hundred, that's what your mother got. Then if your mother loses three hundred species, now you start off at six hundred—half of what your grandmother had. Perhaps it comes as no surprise in this study, the main factor that protected against this generational loss of diversity was adequate prebiotic fiber consumption. Granted, this is just an animal study. But it's impossible to re-create in humans and it really makes sense.

If it seems too good to be true, it might just be that we've been ignoring it

The benefits of postbiotic SCFAs may seem a little too good to be true, but the science is real. SCFAs aren't just important, they're *absolutely vital* to gut health. They offer a solution to dysbiosis by correcting leaky gut and reducing bacterial endotoxemia. They feed and empower the healthy microbes in your gut so they can do their job! They also play a role in human health throughout the entire body. They offer protection from the most deadly diseases in the United States. That by itself should make it the talk of the town, the focus of our national conversation in our quest to better health. Yet this superstar languishes in anonymity. It's time to change that. I'm building a fiber bandwagon. Who's coming with me? Invite your friends. Grab your family. Let's be loud and proud so they can hear us. It's time for us all to be *Fiber Fueled.*

To view the 65⁺ scientific references cited in this chapter, please visit me online at www.theplantfedgut.com/research/.

PART II
THE FIBER FUELED APPROACH

4

Eat the Rainbow to Find Your Pot of Gold

Why diversity of plants should be on your mind every time you eat

Now that we've established the incredible health benefits of being *Fiber Fueled*, it's time to count our daily grams of fiber and load up on Wheaties, Fiber One bars, and Metamucil, right? Not so fast, my friends!

In 2017 I sat in the front row of a jam-packed, standing-room-only lecture in Chicago. It was Digestive Disease Week, the biggest meeting of gastroenterologists, surgeons, nutritionists, and researchers in the world, with close to twenty thousand nerds (like me) from 150 countries. I was there to hear Dr. Rob Knight speak. Dr. Knight is a god of gut health, in my opinion. He created the American Gut Project in 2012, the largest and most diverse study of microbes and microbiomes of the industrialized world. Dr. Knight was at the podium to announce the greatest predictor of a healthy microbiome using the full, unprecedented strength of his American Gut database. An announcement coming from the highest-quality source we have that would redefine how we think of gut health. His finding?

The single greatest predictor of a healthy gut microbiome is the diversity of plants in one's diet.

That's right. Not Metamucil, not simply counting grams of fiber, but the diversity of plants in your diet. More specifically, he found that the consumption of *thirty different plants* in a given week was the greatest predictor of gut microbial diversity. Believe it or not, this was far more powerful than whether you self-identify as "vegan," "vegetarian," or "omnivore." Why? Well, you can be a junk food vegan and eat very few plants and you can eat a Paleo diet that emphasizes plant-based diversity, and this can actually be a healthy diet with the proper modifications. It all comes back to diversity of plants.

Since you've been following along closely, I bet you're not too surprised by this. In Chapter 2 we saw the effects of just five days on a plant-based diet for gut health, which were dramatic when compared to five days on an animal-based diet. We also know from Chapter 3 how important fiber, which is found in plants, is to gut health—specifically how important prebiotic fiber is, because it can be transformed into postbiotic SCFAs by our probiotic gut microbes. And we know that there are innumerable types of fiber in nature, and every plant provides a distinct mix that requires a unique blend of microbes to process it. A diet that maximizes a variety of dietary fibers and resistant starches supports the diverse microbial community that's necessary to process it. As proven by the Hazda population, the more fiber and plant diversity, the more diversity in the microbiota. Why is diversity important? Because the adaptability of our gut microbiota allows us to unlock the healing power of SCFAs. We need a team of microbes to get all the benefits.

Dr. Knight's American Gut Project study also found that people who consumed an increased diversity of plants had a greater representation of SCFA-producing bacteria. Remember in the last chapter when we discussed training your gut with fiber? Regular exercise forces your muscles to adapt and get stronger. Similarly, giving your gut regular practice with fiber increases the representation of fiber-metabolizing, SCFA-producing bugs that are hyperefficient at extracting the SCFAs for you—an adapted, stronger gut, if you will. You get better at things the more you practice, right? Well, so does your gut.

As we know from Chapter 2, the composition of our microbiome is determined in large part by the foods we eat. Dietary choices lead to the rise and fall of microbes within our gut minute by minute. Every single plant type has a community of gut microbes that thrive when that food is present and languish if that food is removed. Therefore, it makes sense that the diversity within our microbiome would be proportional to the diversity of plants in our diet. More plant-based diversity = stronger, healthier microbiota = stronger, healthier you.

Although our food technology continues to rapidly progress and we have increased availability of food, the diversity in our diet is plummeting. There are approximately four hundred thousand varieties of plants on Earth, of which about three hundred thousand are edible. But combined globally we consume only around two hundred species in total. Folks, this means we're eating only one out of every fifteen hundred edible plants on this planet.

Not to mention that just three crops—rice, maize, and wheat—contribute nearly 60 percent of calories and proteins humans obtain from plants. Consolidation in high-yield crops is a lot easier for the food production system than supporting diversity. In the last century alone we've abandoned 75 percent of the plant diversity in our agricultural practices as farmers worldwide have been pressured to use genetically uniform, high-yielding varieties. In other words, our modern food systems are efficiently producing calories at the expense of nutrients and biodiversity.

What this means is that plant-based diversity in your diet will not happen by accident. It happens by making this your core dietary philosophy, shunning the path that our food system wants you to take. The good news is that in the pages that follow I'm going to help you maximize your plant-based diversity as a celebration of nature's bounty.

Plant-based diversity: Make it the golden rule

Plant-based diversity is in fact so powerful, so life- and health-changing, that it should be our Golden Rule of eating. By following the one Golden Rule of healthy eating you can have it all—the flavors, smells, and textures from food that you love, food that also just so happens to bring you more vitality and health rather than taking it away. Food that makes you live longer, look better, and feel better. Food that heals and improves your gut microbiome. Food that makes you feel sexy, look sexy, and want more sexy time. I've lived it first-hand, and I've witnessed it in my patients.

When you maximize plant-based diversity, you make a choice that grants you better health—you choose food that nourishes and sustains your optimal health rather than the foods that zap your energy and beat up your gut microbiota until dysbiosis, the root cause of disease, sets in. By focusing on diversity of plants, you maximize the different nutrients that your food contains to reverse your medical problems and even heal the ones that you don't yet realize exist. And by choosing plant diversity, you are fueling your microbiome with the scientifically proven number one determinant of a healthy gut and unleashing the healing power of SCFAs throughout the entire body.

We've made health too complicated with our extensive lists of foods to avoid, complex percentages of fats-to-protein-to-carb ratios, elimination diets, calorie counting, even weighing our food—and despite all these rules, we're not getting any better. It just doesn't need to be this complicated. Diversity of plants. That's it. That's all you have to remember. Done. No more annoying food lists. If you follow this one rule, it will lead you to better health. And it will always be the truth no matter what happens: No matter what changes on this planet or in our lifestyles, this core tenet of better health will stay the same.

You might be hearing "plant-based diversity" and wondering, "But aren't vegans—who subsist on plant-based protein including lots of beans—suffering from nutrient deficiencies?" One of the big fears with the vegan—or plant-based—diet is that we'll be missing out on critical micronutrients. Rest assured: A 2014 study compared the overall nutritional value of multiple different diets (vegan, vegetarian, semi-vegetarian, pesco-vegetarian, and omnivorous) and found the vegan diet to be the most nutritionally complete while the omnivorous diet received the lowest score.

This approach to eating always delivers beyond expectation—you may do it to fix your diabetes, for example, but along the way you're fixing everything else, too, including the stuff that's not even become a problem yet. The Golden Rule of plant-based diversity is both healing and preventative. It's incredibly powerful.

If you make it your core philosophy for how you choose to eat on a daily basis, this one simple rule will open up a world of possibility for you. No more calorie counting, eating tasteless diet foods, or restricting portion sizes. You can eat as much as you want and still be your ideal body weight and have better health. Let me repeat that: You can eat as much as you want and be your ideal body weight. Yes, I said that. I know this seems like a crazy concept in the context of what's been dominating our health and diet culture for decades, but it's real and it works. If you think about all the herbs, flavors, textures, and varieties of health-promoting plant food that you can eat without restriction— that's wild. And so exciting!

Every plant has its own unique mix of gut-healing fiber

- Barley has a prebiotic fiber called beta-glucan that promotes the growth of healthy microbes, lowers total and LDL cholesterol, and helps regulate blood sugar. On a side note, barley is also rich in selenium, which is important for thyroid health and may prevent autoimmune thyroid disease.

- Whole oats are also high in beta-glucan. In addition, oats have phenolic acids that offer antioxidant and anti-inflammatory protection as a bonus.

- Flaxseeds are 20 to 40 percent soluble prebiotic fiber from mucilage gums, which give you blissful bowel movements. They also kick your gut microbes into high gear. I have more love for flaxseeds, so we'll come back to them later.

- Wheat bran has a special type of fiber made of arabinoxylan oligosaccharides shown to boost healthy gut microbes like *Bifidobacteria* and reduce digestive symptoms like flatulence and abdominal pain. It also has antioxidant and anticancer effects. One of the great scientists of our generation, Dr. Balfour Sartor at the University of North Carolina, has been touting the benefits of bran for years, even when others were criticizing wheat. Bran is the hard outer coating that protects the seed and is often removed in food processing. So if you're choosing refined grains or are unnecessarily gluten-free, you won't get to enjoy these benefits. We'll talk more about gluten later in this chapter. I know you're wondering.

- White potatoes are an excellent source of resistant starch. That's right: white potatoes. French fries and potato chips are obviously bad but my Irish microbes love a good potato mash. They're a great source of prebiotic resistant starch! In one study, they increased SCFA levels more than inulin from chicory root. Here's a tip: If you let your potatoes cool, the process of cooling creates more resistant starch. If you heat and cool repeatedly, you just keep turning it up. Leftover mashed potatoes, anyone?

- Seaweed! Seaweed rocks fiber content that is 50 to 85 percent soluble prebiotic. It may explain some of the longevity seen in Japan, where it's regularly consumed. I'll talk more about seaweed in Chapter 8. It's a great addition to a *Fiber Fueled* diet.

Phytochemicals: Game changers beyond fiber

Each plant offers you a unique mix of nutrients: fiber, plant protein, carbohydrates, healthy fats, vitamins, minerals, and so on. We have talked a lot about fiber, but the benefits of phytochemicals shouldn't be overlooked. "Phyto-" is a prefix meaning "plant." Phytochemicals are exclusive nutrients that you'll only find in plant foods, and there are at least 8,000 of them, most of which we know very little about. Only about 150 of them have actually been studied. But what we keep finding, study after study, is that phytochemicals are good for us.

Let me give you an example. People say, "An apple a day keeps the doctor away." Could this old adage possibly be true? Recent studies emphatically say, "Yes!" No surprise, apples are a great source of fiber. A medium-size apple has 4.4 grams of fiber, about two-thirds insoluble and one-third soluble fiber. That's just the beginning. Apples also contain numerous phytochemicals. Quercetin-3-galactoside, quercetin-3-glucoside, quercetin-3-rhamnoside, catechin, epicatechin, procyanidin, cyanidin-3-galactoside, coumaric acid, chlorogenic acid, gallic acid, and phloridzin—to name just a few. Each part of the apple has a different mix of phytochemicals, depending on whether you're looking at the peel, the pulp, or even the core.

Each of these phytochemicals has unique healing properties. For example, quercetin protects against lung and colon cancer, coronary artery disease, type 2 diabetes, asthma, and liver damage. Catechins protect against lung cancer, coronary artery disease, stroke, and chronic obstructive pulmonary disease.

And did you know apples have probiotics? Put down the capsule and pick up an apple because a single apple may contain as many as one hundred million bacteria. Plants have a microbiome, too! Just like in humans, the microbes contribute greatly to the health and development of the apple from flower to fruit. The apple has tremendous diversity, with literally thousands of species. In fact, organically produced apples have not only more microbial diversity, but they also have a shift toward higher levels of microbes known to have a benefit on human health, such as the probiotic *Lactobacilli*. Scientists now believe that this exchange between the plant microbiome and the human gut microbiome may be of special importance for human health and a crucial source of microbes for our gut. It is yet another example of how we're all a part of the circle of life, and everything in our universe is interconnected.

Not every apple is the same. We now see that each varietal has its own unique mix of health-promoting stuff. But in all cases the fiber, phytochemicals, and microbes contribute in some way to human health. This explains why apples have been found to reduce the risk of developing cancer, heart disease, asthma, and type 2 diabetes.

So should we all gorge ourselves on a bushel of apples daily? Absolutely not. This is just a window into the magic of fruits and vegetables. Apples are one fruit, and I share this case study with you to show you some of the amazing qualities you'll find in apples. But every single fruit, vegetable, whole grain, legume, seed, and nut has its own unique blend of fiber, phytochemicals, and microbes worthy of a celebration.

Many of the colors that you see in plants are the result of their phytochemicals. So when you hear people saying, "Eat the rainbow," this is the reason why. It's top secret code for "Diversity of Plants."

BENEFITS OF EATING THE RAINBOW

COLOR	PLANT	PHYTOCHEMICALS	BENEFITS
Red	Tomatoes, watermelon	Lycopene	Provides antioxidants; protects against prostate cancer
Orange	Carrots, sweet potatoes, pumpkins	Beta-carotene	Supports healthy skin, immune system, and eyes

COLOR	PLANT	PHYTOCHEMICALS	BENEFITS
Yellow-orange	Oranges, lemons, peaches	Limonoids, flavonoids	Protects against cancer and heart disease
Green	Spinach, kale, collards	Chlorophyll, lutein	Protects against cancer; protects healthy eyes
Green-white	Broccoli, Brussels sprouts, cabbage, cauliflower	Indoles, isothiocyanates	Very strong cancer protection
White-green	Garlic, onions, chives, asparagus	Allyl sulfides	Lowers cholesterol and blood pressure, reduces risk of stomach cancer and heart disease
Blue	Blueberries, blackberries	Anthocyanins	Provides antioxidants, improves memory, protects against cancer
Purple	Purple grapes, plums	Resveratrol	Lowers cholesterol, protects against clots
Brown	Whole grains, legumes	Fiber!	Read Chapter 3!

It gets better. Two different plants can create a synergistic effect—it's like nature's version of a match made in heaven. For example:

- **Tomatoes and avocadoes in guacamole:** Tomatoes are rich in lycopene, which reduces cancer risk and cardiovascular disease. Healthy fats from avocadoes make the lycopene more bioavailable. Yay healthy fats!
- **A mixed fruit bowl:** A study out of Cornell University discovered that combinations of fruit resulted in greater antioxidant activity that was additive and synergistic. Based upon this, the authors recommended "that to improve their nutrition and health, consumers should be getting antioxidants from a diverse diet."

- **Kale and lemon:** Kale is a plant-based source of iron, which is non-heme and less bioavailable. Heme iron comes from animal products, is more bioavailable, but also more inflammatory and has been associated with coronary artery disease, colon cancer, and type 2 diabetes. The vitamin C from a lemon cranks up iron absorption and allows you to get what you need from a non–heart disease/colon cancer/diabetes-inducing source, meaning a plant.
- **Turmeric and black pepper:** The active ingredient in turmeric is curcumin, a potent anti-inflammatory that actually works great for people with joint pains. By sprinkling black pepper on your curry, you increase the bioavailability of curcumin by 2,000 percent.

Picture sitting down at every meal and eating food that you absolutely love. Your plate is full of color—bright greens and reds, soothing blues and purple, sunny yellow and orange. All the flavors are there—sweet, salty, bitter, sour, and umami (savory). The smells are simply divine, conjuring up memories of the best homemade meal you ever had, making your belly feel warm and your mouth start to water. There are tons of variation in texture, with crunch balanced against soft and chewy. And when you're done eating, you feel fantastic. No food hangover that requires a bolus of caffeine to compensate for it. You feel energized and light—your very best self. How liberating would it be for you to enjoy a meal like that without worrying about compliance with complex rules or food lists, to be driven instead by color and taste and texture.

This is the life I envision for you. It's vibrantly colorful. It's fun and fresh. It's effortlessly healthy. Plant-based diversity is the antithesis of categorical food restriction. There's been a trend toward deeper and deeper food restrictions out there, but it's not working because the true solution is radical abundance, not extreme deprivation. With that in mind, I want to walk you through the science behind some of the targets of dietary restriction and show you that we're better with these foods back in our lives.

The power of whole grains

Many of us have been led to believe that whole grains are inflammatory and that they are an unhealthy product of modern agriculture; this belief makes me cringe. We really shouldn't be lumping whole grains in with refined grains, like sugar. They're totally different. Whole grains are an excellent source of prebiotic fiber and definitely belong in a diet that's rich in plant-based diversity. If you're skeptical, allow me to share some of the research.

In a systematic review and meta-analysis of forty-five studies, increasing your daily whole-grain consumption by just two pieces of whole-grain bread rewarded the participants with a reduced risk of coronary heart disease, cardiovascular disease, and total cancer as well as a lower likelihood of death from all causes, respiratory diseases, infectious diseases, diabetes, and all non-cardiovascular, non-cancer causes. Convinced yet?

I'll give you more: In a meta-analysis of the Nurses' Health Study and the Health Professionals Follow-Up Study they found that every daily serving of whole grains reduces your risk of death by 5 percent and your risk of death by cardiovascular cause by 9 percent.

- In another meta-analysis including nearly 250,000 people, those eating the most whole grains had a 14 percent lower risk of stroke than those eating the fewest.
- A 2011 meta-analysis of prospective studies found that there was a 20 percent reduction in the risk of colorectal cancer for every three servings of whole grains consumed per day, and the risk was even lower with higher intakes.

- Another meta-analysis, this time with fifteen studies and almost 120,000 people, found that eating three servings of whole grains daily was linked to lower body mass index and less belly fat.
- A systematic review and meta-analysis of sixteen cohort studies found that eating at least three servings of whole grains per day could lower your risk of diabetes by a third! There was no such benefit from eating refined grains, by the way. In fact, whole-grain bread, whole-grain cereals, wheat bran, and brown rice were all found to be protective on sub-analysis, while white rice actually increased risk.

I can't write a gut health book without showing you what happens to your microbes when you consume whole grains. In a randomized controlled trial, study subjects who substituted whole grains for refined grains saw growth of SCFA-producing bacteria *Lachnospira*, increased SCFA levels, and a decrease in pro-inflammatory *Enterobacteriaceae*. They also noted improvement in the immune system and no effect on gut inflammation. In other words, whole grains were good for the gut. You may recall from Chapter 2 that the long-term adherence to a Paleolithic diet made the gut microbiota less healthy, with more TMAO and fewer SCFAs, which the authors attributed to the elimination of whole grains from the diet.

How about inflammation? Do whole grains cause inflammation? In a randomized controlled crossover study, those consuming whole grains saw their measure of inflammation, the C-reactive protein, drop by 21 percent while those who eliminated whole grains saw theirs increase by 12 percent. In a ten-year study of dietary patterns, whole-grain consumption had the *strongest* anti-inflammatory effect of the thirty-seven food groups studied. The evidence is clear: Whole grains are anti-inflammatory.

When we discuss carbohydrates, let's separate destructive, refined grains from the health-promoting whole grains. Whole grains are a great source of the fiber that we read about in Chapter 3, empowering our microbes, and releasing SCFAs that protect us against obesity, heart disease, stroke, and type 2 diabetes. Whole grains aren't inflammatory; they're quite the opposite. If you want to villainize "carbs," do it to the refined grains and leave the microbiota-supporting, health-producing whole grains alone!

But what about gluten?

There has been so much talk about gluten in recent years, so let's get into it. Gluten is a protein found in three specific whole grains: wheat, barley, and rye. And, of course, it's in any products that include wheat, barley, and rye. Since most of us have never even seen raw wheat, it's fair to acknowledge that almost all gluten-containing foods *are* processed foods—bread, pasta, pizza, and cereal. And that, my friends, is one of the main reasons that people may feel better when they go gluten-free. The elimination of ultra-processed foods, including refined carbs, is something that I support 100 percent. But does it make sense to categorically eliminate *all* gluten-containing products, or are we throwing the baby out with the bathwater?

Gluten is a problem for people with celiac disease. They need to be completely gluten-free and there's no debate. But there's the perception by some that gluten is inflammatory, causes leaky gut and autoimmune disease, and that we should all be gluten-free. It's a growing trend that started with a bunch of test-tube studies and has snowballed to this place where a third of Americans are actively restricting gluten intake. If these test-tube studies are correct and gluten really does cause leaky gut, then we should see improvements in gut health with a gluten-free diet, right?

But we don't. We actually see the opposite. After healthy subjects without celiac spent a month on a gluten-free diet, counts of healthy bacteria like *F. prausnitzii*, *Lactobacillus*, and *Bifidobacterium* declined while evildoers *E. coli* and *Enterobacteriaceae* increased.

In a randomized, controlled crossover study, a "low gluten" diet reduced healthy *Bifidobacterium* and butyrate-producing *Anaerostipes hadrus* and *Eubacterium hallii*. I know you're still wondering whether gluten causes inflammation, affects the immune system, even causes increased intestinal permeability. When researchers tested humans, they couldn't find any evidence of inflammation, immune activation, or increased intestinal permeability connected to the consumption of gluten in this study. But there was a difference in immune reactivity in a test tube. As I've mentioned before, laboratory tests don't always translate to human studies.

In another study, whole wheat increased healthy *Bifidobacterium* and produced metabolites that *improved* intestinal integrity and *reduced* intestinal permeability. Let me say that again—whole wheat *improved* intestinal integrity and *reduced* intestinal permeability (or leaky gut).

What we're seeing here is the difference between laboratory and human research. In the lab, you may extract the molecule of interest then study it in isolation, often in a concentrated form in a test tube. Clearly, this is quite different from when a human being actually eats a gluten-containing food in real life. For me, I take those laboratory studies with a major grain of salt and have more trust in the human studies that show us what happens in a natural setting. As you've seen, when healthy people eat wheat or other gluten-containing foods, we find that their gut actually appears more healthy. We've also seen that a gluten-free or restricted diet appears to diminish the SCFA-producing microbes and to enhance the inflammatory ones.

There's more fallout from going gluten-free. A "low-gluten" diet causes loss of the genes for carbohydrate metabolism. Back in Chapter 3 we mentioned that we humans only have seventeen glycoside hydrolases, our digestive enzymes for complex carbohydrates. Meanwhile, our gut microbes may have sixty thousand or more of these enzymes. By depriving ourselves of gluten, we actually lose part of that carbohydrate-processing mechanism. So now the gut is weaker and less adapted to processing and unpacking complex carbs; as a result, when you try to reintroduce complex carbs in the future, you struggle. Hello, food sensitivity!

And last but not least, when we eliminate gluten from our diet, the big question is what do we replace it with? We've already discussed the importance of whole grains, and gluten-containing foods are the principal source of whole grains in the American diet. In a prospective cohort study of 6,500 people over 2,273,931 person-years, they found that as people consumed more gluten, their risk of ischemic heart disease *decreased*, which they attributed to the whole grains in gluten-containing foods. In other words, if you cut gluten out, you are increasing your risk of ischemic heart disease, our number one killer. It's worth noting that this is the complete opposite of people who have celiac disease, where the consumption of gluten sets off an inflammatory cascade that may increase their risk of heart disease.

I'll admit, gluten is not a simple topic. That's why you need someone like me, who is qualified and has thoroughly reviewed the science, to give you insights on the right choice for you. In Chapter 5 I will walk you through my gluten protocol to determine whether or not you should continue to consume gluten. Here's a preview: Most of you should! But by no means am I advocating that you make gluten the centerpiece of your diet. I am advocating, however, for plant-based diversity, and to not exclude health-promoting foods from your diet because when you narrow the spectrum of plants in your diet, you also narrow the diversity of your microbiome. And this is true even with wheat.

Legumes: Small in stature, huge on gut-healing fiber!

The average American eats just 6.3 pounds of beans per year. That's down by 20 percent compared to fifty years ago. And yet some argue that legumes are the cause of every modern epidemic, which couldn't be further from the truth. Legumes are jam-packed with fiber. A cup of green peas, for example, has 7 grams of fiber. A cup of lentils? A whopping 16 grams. Pinto beans have 30 grams of fiber per cup.

It's true that the flip side of all that fiber is that consuming an excessive amount of beans can be hard to tolerate for some. But the benefits of legumes can't be argued. Excess weight melts away when you eat a diet high in legumes. Your waist gets smaller. Your blood pressure and cholesterol drop to the point of tapering your drug. Your blood sugar balances and the diabetes disappears. And your risk for having a heart attack or developing colon cancer just got chopped in half.

There are literally hundreds of studies to support beans. Let me share just one example. In a randomized, controlled trial of a legume-packed diet versus legume-free, the researchers held the number of calories constant so that it was about nutrients and not calories. What they saw in the legume group was shocking. The C-reactive protein, a marker of inflammation, dropped by 40 percent. Blood pressure and cholesterol both dropped. But what was most fascinating is that the legume group lost more weight even though they ate the same number of calories. You may recall from Chapter 1 when we discussed that your gut microbiome plays a huge role in weight control, and that it's more than just calories in–calories out.

Should you be eating soy?

There's been some debate about soy due to the perception of its carrying estrogen, but I want you to understand that phytoestrogens aren't estrogen, nor do they act like human estrogen. Instead, phytoestrogens are isoflavones, one of the unique phytochemicals in soy beans. There are actually three soy isoflavones: genistein, daidzein, and glycitein. They have a number of health benefits, including: lowering cholesterol, strengthening bones, treating menopausal symptoms, lowering risk of coronary heart disease, and reducing risk of prostate/colon/breast/ovarian cancers.

Want even more good news about soy? There are certain gut bacteria that can convert soy isoflavones into an even more beneficial compound called equol. This is like a supercharged isoflavone, giving you even more cardiovascular, bone, and menopausal health benefits. Unfortunately, you need to have the bacteria in order to do this. Equol can be produced by 50 to 60 percent of Asian people but just 30 percent of Westerners. For what it's worth, diets high in carbohydrates (really meaning fiber) and low in saturated fat are associated with equol production, while antibiotics appear to hinder it.

I recommend consuming only non-GMO and organic soy in its whole-foods forms: edamame, tofu, miso, tempeh, tamari, and unsweetened soy milk. Model your soy consumption after the way they do it in Asia. For some delicious ways to consume soy, check out the recipes in Chapter 10.

So how about the effect of legumes on the gut microbiota? In a mouse model, both navy beans and black beans increased numbers of beneficial SCFA-producing bacteria with coinciding increased SCFA production, promoted colonic barrier integrity, and reduced bacterial endotoxin levels.

In a randomized crossover study, chickpea consumption for three weeks in addition to their regular diet led to increased growth of SCFA-producing bacteria (*Faecalibacterium prausnitzii*) and decreased growth of the pathogenic and putrefactive bacteria (*Clostridium histolyticum* and *C. lituseburense*). The authors concluded that chickpeas "have the potential to modulate the intestinal microbial composition to promote intestinal health in humans."

Pea protein has been shown to stimulate the growth of the health-promoting bacteria *Lactobacilli* and *Bifidobacteria*. There was a corresponding shift in the bacterial metabolites with increased levels of the short-chain fatty acids (SCFAs). The authors concluded, "Such changes in microbial composition may beneficially impact the intestinal environment and exert a health-promoting effect in humans."

Fascinating, right? So when you take all of this together it comes as no surprise that in a major study of food-intake patterns from around the world there was one—and only one—food shown to make people live longer . . . LEGUMES!

What about lectins?

What are lectins? Well, lectins aren't just one thing; they're actually a large family of protein compounds found in nature that are known because they bind carbohydrates. They're ubiquitous in nature—humans, animals, plants, fungi, and microorganisms all have them. You'll find varying amount of lectins in different foods. Some foods that contain higher amounts of lectins include cow's milk, eggs, beans, peanuts, lentils, tomatoes, potatoes, eggplant, fruits, wheat, and other grains.

In recent years there's been a growing perception that lectins are inflammatory; specifically, that they damage the lining of your gut and over-activate your immune system—and as a result, the thinking goes, lectins may be contributing to our twenty-first-century epidemics. According to this line of argument, the way to counter this is to reduce or eliminate all grains (including pseudo-grains), beans and legumes, nuts, fruits, and many vegetables—massive, in some cases categorical, elimination. But is it justified?

The idea that lectins may cause disease isn't very novel. It has floated around in fringe medical literature for decades based on test-tube and animal-model studies mostly from the 1970s and

1980s. If you only present those studies, lectins can sound very scary.

But there's a reason that well-respected journals and the world's leading doctors and nutritionists aren't cringing in fear from lectins or shying away from beans and grains. First, there's the other side of the story, which is that lectins from wheat, fava beans, soybeans, mushrooms, bananas, buckwheat, and jackfruit have all been implicated as protective against cancer. But more important, experts know that test-tube and animal studies often don't translate well into real life. Similar to our studies on gluten, we need to confirm the findings in human populations. Otherwise we run the risk of finding some pretty quacky things that mislead us and in some cases can harm us.

So what do we find when we study legumes and whole grains in human populations? Well, you already know. Weight loss. Lower blood pressure and lower cholesterol. Reversal of insulin resistance. Less inflammation. A shift in the microbiome to produce more SCFAs. Protection from cardiovascular disease and cancer. Longer life expectancy. Study after study has shown us that legumes and whole grains are absolutely vital to your health and your gut's health. They're a powerful source of fiber and their unique qualities make them irreplaceable if you eliminate them. Remember: What's the single greatest predictor of a healthy gut microbiome? The diversity of plants in your diet.

Let's talk about legumes and grains *together* for a minute. Did you know that when you combine beans with a whole grain, you create a complete protein package, ramp up the fiber, and get your protein from a low-calorie, high-nutrient plant source? Remember, the source of our protein matters, and when you replace animal protein with plant sources you find that people are healthier and live longer. Consider that Costa Rica outperforms the United States in life expectancy on a diet centered around beans and rice while spending a mere fraction on health care. They're not the only ones! Legumes and whole grains are celebrated in the diets of all five Blue Zones. These are longevity foods, and they are the foundation of gut health.

It all comes back to the Golden Rule—Diversity of Plants!

Would you agree that a healthy diet is one that maximizes nutrients in terms of achieving optimal amounts for bodily function? This is the concept of "nutrient density," meaning that we want as many nutrients as possible per calorie that we consume. But nutrient density alone just isn't enough to describe an ideal diet. What if you ate kale, and kale only, all day long, and nothing else. Would you be healthy?

Absolutely not. Kale is a superfood, but if it's the only thing you ate you'd be redundantly and excessively loading up on the nutrients that kale provides but missing out on the nutrients, fiber variety, and microbes you'd get from other plants. For example, if you consumed 2,000 calories of kale per day you'd get 30 times more copper, 80 times more vitamin A, 80 times more vitamin C, and 360 times more vitamin K than you actually need. Hopefully you just urinate it out, but there comes a point for anything in life where too much of a good thing can actually be harmful. Meanwhile you'd be sorely missing the lycopene that you find in tomatoes, the selenium you find in Brazil nuts, and the vitamin B$_5$ from avocados. Eventually those nutrient deficiencies set in. You'd get nearly 150 grams of fiber per day, but it would all be of the same type. No diversity of plants to provide diversity of fiber to a diversity of microbes. You would miss out on all the other species you'd find in the microbiota of other plant foods.

We have a tendency in our culture to obsess over superfoods. Like the celebrities of food, we put them on a pedestal and celebrate their elite nutrient density and special properties. I'm going to give you some of my favorites in Chapter 8, and they're foods that are dear to my heart. But if you ate *only* the foods in Chapter 8, your diet wouldn't be as healthy as the person who's just really good at maximizing plant-based diversity in their diet. In my program, I focus on maximizing plant-based diversity first, and then incorporate superfoods.

To recap:

Every time you go to the supermarket: Think *Diversity of Plants!*
Every time you're cooking a meal: *Diversity of Plants!*
When you sit down at the dinner table and start loading up your plate: *Diversity of Plants!*

As a medical doctor, I know when someone is actively dying, even if they're still alive. You see how one organ affects the other. When one fails, it drags down another, setting off a chain reaction that leads to multi-organ failure and ultimate demise. What if we could do the opposite of this, and simultaneously lift all organs up at once? With a plant-centered diet, you're not just fixing one problem, you are fixing *all of them* and optimizing the health of your organs in the process. Not just treating disease, not just avoiding disease, but actually optimizing your body and making it better. Becoming your best self.

Eating a diet fully enriched with all the colors, flavors, and nutrients nature has to offer is all you need. Remember the Golden Rule that will never change:

Diversity of Plants, Diversity of Plants, Diversity of Plants.

To view the 45+ scientific references cited in this chapter, please visit me online at www.theplantfedgut.com/research/.

5

Finding Your Plant Passion with a Sensitive Gut
Your custom plan to ease bloating, gas, cramps, and altered bowels

*I*suspect that many of you are thinking right now, *How am I going to do this? I feel horrible when I eat those foods. What if my body hates fiber?* Statistically that's 15 to 20 percent of people, but since you're reading this book, there's a decent chance you have irritable bowel. Fifty to 80 percent of people with IBS have food sensitivities. But you are the person who needs this book the most. That's the great irony. The people who need fiber the most are the ones who will also struggle the most to eat it. You have to fix the gut to reap the reward of better health. And to fix the gut, we know we need fiber and diversity of plants.

So what does it say that you struggle to process fiber or certain types of plants? Well, it indicates that your gut has been damaged. Of course people with digestive disorders are going to struggle more with these foods. But it's not just them. This may also be true for people with allergic and immune system disorders. Or migraines, anxiety, or depression, or, frankly, any of the litany of conditions that we learned is associated with dysbiosis in Chapter 1. Where there's dysbiosis you'll also find food sensitivities. If that's you, then I want to help you the most because then we are correcting the root cause of your problem *and* helping you enjoy your food again.

That doesn't mean it's going to be easy. You've been searching for solutions to your problem and the solution that's been offered to you for the last fifteen years has been, "Well just get rid of it." And when you do this, you may feel better in the short term. But are you better in the long term? Generally not. Elimination, particularly categorical elimination, is short-term gain and long-term pain.

It's clear that the Golden Rule is in direct conflict with the idea of eliminating entire plant categories. We learned in Chapter 4 that when you eliminate plant categories you deprive yourself of the health benefits and alter the balance of bacteria in your gut to favor dysbiosis.

So why do people do it? Why do people eliminate beans, grains, and nightshades?

Part of the reason is that many of these foods bring out the worst in their gut—gas, bloating, cramping pain, and weird noises. I'm sure you've seen the photos on the internet that show a protuberant, pregnancy-like belly and a flat belly from the exact same day. I can't tell you how many patients have brought these photos to my office as evidence of a problem. They're not as helpful as the poop selfies, but I understand that you want to show that something is wrong.

The thing is that these symptoms of digestive distress have been, unfortunately, misinterpreted. I see a lot of people on the Internet, even some medical doctors, claiming that bloating and gas brought on by plant foods means that they're inflammatory. But as we discussed in Chapter 4, these foods have repeatedly proven to be the opposite—*anti*-inflammatory. I've also taken care of plenty of patients who think that because they have these symptoms it means they're incapable of eating these foods, and therefore it makes sense to acknowledge the problem, eliminate the triggers, and move on.

But think of it this way: If you have arthritis in your knee, does that mean you should buy a motorized scooter and stop walking? Sure, if you quit walking, you'll never feel that discomfort in your knee again, right? But then your exercise falls off, your legs atrophy, you gain weight, then end up on multiple medications to control your blood pressure/cholesterol/diabetes, and you feel depressed and weak. But hey, your knee doesn't hurt! Is that worth it?

If, instead, you put in the effort and decide, *I'm going to walk, do some physical therapy, exercise my leg and knee*, then you'll actually be able to lessen the pain and at the same time maintain health throughout your body. For the person with arthritis, it's painful in the beginning to start healing through exercise and therapy. But weathering that initial discomfort, the reward is a stronger knee, increased functional capacity, and better health that extends beyond the knee. The same is true with food sensitivities—if you accept that while it may not be easy in the short term, it's so much better in the long term, we can work through the short-term effects together. The point is that there will be unintended consequences when we allow unhealthy lifestyle habits to form. But there's also the flip side, which are the unintended benefits that come when we choose health and opt for plant-based diversity.

In the coming pages I'll break down the science behind why people develop food sensitivities and lay out our plan to address them. If you take it slow and take your time adding in plant-based foods, you'll reach the long-term reward for short-term discomfort: a stronger gut, broader plant-based diversity, and better health that extends beyond the belly.

Share the Message

There are so many other people who need to hear the message of plant-based diversity for gut health. I mean, I wish I could go back to the younger version of myself and slap this book across my head. Softcover version, of course. I wouldn't have wasted all those years feeling miserable. So what I'm saying is that you, too, can be a transformative power for positive change. This book is nothing if it sits on the shelf. NOTHING. But this is something really powerful in the hands of a reader, and if you've felt that power, share it with others. Discuss it, recommend it, share your copy, gift it, send them to the library, post your favorite piece of knowledge to social media. We all can do our part to promote consciousness in our food choices and help people heal. Just think of what you've accomplished by getting one person to read this book and transform their health! We can all be instruments of change for a better world.

Why do we get food sensitivities? Why not with meat?

It's your gut microbiota! When you curse the heavens as you watch your friend scarf down unlimited quantities of that six-bean chili while you try to maintain a straight face and not show the discomfort you're experiencing, just know . . . it's not you. It's your bugs. Yes, you are 99.9 percent genetically the same as that person sitting across from you. But your gut microbiome is a totally different story, completely uniquely yours. It's just as personal as your fingerprint. There is literally no one on the planet with a gut microbiome exactly like yours. If you had an identical twin, you'd most closely resemble your twin followed by your mother, yet still be entirely distinct.

Your unique gut microbiome has strengths and weaknesses that are uniquely yours. It may be really good at processing beans but really struggle with garlic and onions. In a perfect world, if your diet perfectly complemented the strengths and weaknesses of your gut, then you wouldn't have any food sensitivity at all. None.

Since your diet and your microbiome are completely intertwined, your diet needs to be just as personal to you as your microbiome is.

You need to use some trial and error to discover your custom, ideal diet. Now it may seem contradictory to say "There's no one size fits all" immediately after defining "one Golden Rule for better health." But it's rather simple: You follow the Golden Rule of maximizing diversity of plants with every meal, but recognize that how that looks for you is going to be different from the person sitting next to you who is eating from the same selection of foods.

The goal is to hit that sweet spot where your dietary choices are perfectly matched to the strengths and weaknesses of your gut, and then magic ensues. No digestive distress, maximum plants, healing gut and body. We're going to help you identify some of the strengths and weaknesses in your gut so that we can get started fine-tuning, not by eliminating foods but by going slow. We're going to get you to that sweet spot.

The important thing to remember is that it's not about perfection. And yes, there will be times when you'll have gas, bloating, discomfort, or altered bowels. We all have that from time to time, myself included. But what we are going to do is optimize your gut and, in doing so, make those symptoms infrequent to the point that they no longer command your attention or affect your quality of life.

The way we accomplish this is by treating your gut like a muscle. Every time you sit down to eat it's like your gut is going to the gym. Physical fitness is defined by health and well-being achieved through nutrition, exercise, and sufficient rest to optimize performance in some way, whether it's sports or just activities of daily living. If our gut is a muscle, gut fitness means digestive health fueled by fiber and achieved by training your gut through plant-based diversity.

In the gym, if you always work out your biceps but never work out your triceps, you're going to have some unbalanced, funny-looking arms. If you don't work out a muscle group, it atrophies. If you don't use it, you lose it, right? Same rules apply to the gut. If you eliminate a food group, your ability to consume that food dwindles.

What if you've been out of commission for a few months due to an injury? If you go to the gym and try to lift three hundred pounds on your first day, you're going to hurt yourself. In the same regard, if you haven't been eating beans and you scarf down a big bowl of the six-bean chili, you're going to feel it because your body isn't adapted or trained for what you're doing.

So what's the best approach in the gym? Work out every single muscle group, just enough to promote growth without injury, and often enough to keep them all maintained or growing. This is exactly the way we should handle our food. We need to work out our gut with every plant category, just enough without overdoing it, and often enough to build our tolerance. Think of every single plant variety as working out a different muscle group. By emphasizing diversity of plants, you are giving your gut the dynamic workout that it's craving. So all plant groups need to be on the menu from time to time, not necessarily daily but often enough to maintain our gut fitness.

We all know the building block of muscle. It's the thing we're getting too much of yet still worry it's not enough—protein. But if we're treating the gut like a muscle, we should recognize the building block of that muscle—fiber. You can't build a healthy gut without fiber.

And here's what's cool: Just like with exercise, your gut will get stronger and become better adapted to what you're trying to do. That's a big takeaway from this book. Your gut is adaptable, and it will adjust to your choices.

Consider this example: Remember in Chapter 2 when we discussed the modern-day hunter-gatherer Hadza tribe of Tanzania? They consume more than 100 grams of fiber per day, about six hundred varieties of plants per year, and have 40 percent more gut diversity than the average American. It turns out that there's a seasonal variation to how they eat that causes a seasonal change in their microbiota. In the wet season, which lasts from November to April, they're more likely to forage for berries. During the dry season from May to October, they hunt animals. Meanwhile, year-round they consume tubers and a variety of plants to get 100 grams of fiber or more per day.

When researchers studied the microbiome of the Hazda, they saw that many species of bacteria disappear for a season and then reappear. And the functional ability of their microbiome alters as a result. Researchers found that foods eaten more regularly resulted in enrichment of the enzymes necessary to digest them. In the wet season when the Hadza consume more berries, they noticed enrichment of the enzymes needed to process a specific component of the berries called fructans. Sear that last sentence into your brain because we're going to come back to it in a moment.

Here's another example: Consider lactose, a short-chain carbohydrate (or sugar) found in dairy products. When I use the term "sugar" here, I don't mean table sugar or glucose, but rather I'm referring to a simple carbohydrate, as opposed to fiber or starch. In order for lactose to be processed we need the enzyme lactase. But 75 percent of the world's population are deficient in this enzyme, and therefore lactose intolerant. So three in four people have the potential for gas, bloating, digestive distress, and altered bowel habits if they consume dairy.

But can people make themselves *less* lactose intolerant? Is it possible to train the gut to handle lactose?

First of all, there is an amount of lactose that can be tolerated in these cases. If I take a medicine dropper and put two drops of cow's milk on someone's tongue, they're not going to have blow-out explosive diarrhea from that. No one is *that* lactose intolerant. So there's a threshold that needs to be crossed to trigger the symptoms.

Second, the gut adapts to regular exposure to lactose. For example, regular consumption of lactose over the course of ten days led to adaptation of colonic bacteria with more lactase activity, less digestive distress, and objectively far less production of gas. In another study, ten days of regular lactose consumption led to improved efficiency of lactose digestion and reduced gas production by threefold.

What does this all mean? First, there is a threshold of tolerance that exists and if we cross that threshold we get symptoms but if we stay within the bounds we should be feeling pretty good. Second, your gut adapts to what you give it. In other words, your gut can be trained to tolerate foods that you're sensitive to. Third, your gut needs to be fed in order to be trained. In other words, elimination diets will only heighten food sensitivities.

Got Milk?

For the record, you shouldn't. I am not advocating for training your gut to handle lactose. We learned about the effect of animal protein and saturated fat on the gut in Chapter 2—less SCFA-producing bacteria, more inflammatory bacteria, increased TMAO production, increased intestinal permeability, and increases in bacterial endotoxin. As we've done in the past, when we examine the whole food rather than a sum of its parts, we find that dairy products have been associated with prostate cancer and Parkinson's disease. Also the link to bone health turns out to be a myth—a prospective study of ninety-six thousand people over twenty-two years showed that milk consumption during teenage years did not protect against hip fracture later in life. In fact, men who drank more milk as a teenager actually had increased risk of hip fracture in the study. In a study of women in Sweden, high milk intake was associated with increased risk of bone fracture, heart disease, cancer, and premature death. One of the first things I do with my patients who have gas, bloating, or diarrhea is to eliminate dairy. You would not believe how many of them are cured just by doing this. Sorry, but milk doesn't do a body good. The irony is that lactose, which has been vilified through the years as evil, is probably the most redeeming thing about dairy because lactose is actually a prebiotic and can have a beneficial effect on the gut microbiota.

Let's take a step back for a moment. Remember in Chapter 3 when we discussed that we humans only have seventeen of the carbohydrate-processing enzymes called glycoside hydrolases? Meanwhile, our gut bacteria have been estimated to have as many as sixty thousand of these digestive enzymes! What this means is we've outsourced carbohydrate processing. Why? Because it makes us adaptable to a variable diet and environment.

It also means that carbohydrate processing—including fiber—requires a healthy, properly adapted gut microbiome. When we damage the gut and reduce diversity, we also reduce the number and types of digestive enzymes in our gut. And that is the reason why there are so many people struggling to deal with carbs these days. We're not eating enough of them to train our gut, and then we're damaging our gut with the other aspects of our lifestyle—processed food, meat and dairy, antibiotics, medications, hypersterility, and sedentarism.

The irony is that we need complex carbohydrates in our diet . . . terribly. They're our prebiotic foods. That's how we *Fiber Fuel* our body and reap the healing benefits of SCFAs. So there is this vicious cycle where complex carbs cause digestive distress, which motivates us to reduce our intake or, worse yet, eliminate them, which weakens the microbiome and makes it less capable of processing carbs so that next time you try them your digestive distress is even worse. So then we label all carbs as being inflammatory and bad for us when in fact they're actually the solution. It's a common mistake that's been prescribed by numerous fad diets, and at best it's short-term gain with long-term loss.

A closer look at inflammatory foods in the gut

Studies keep showing that the complex carbohydrates you'll find in whole fruits, veggies, legumes, and whole grains are anything but inflammatory. They're actually anti-inflammatory. But we rely on our gut microbiome to process them, and if there's damage to the gut then it's also impaired in carbohydrate processing, which leads to digestive distress. That's not inflammation, that's just sloppy processing. It doesn't hurt you beyond the acute symptoms. But what does hurt you is the effect that you see from animal product consumption—less SCFA-producing good bacteria, more inflammatory bacteria, increased intestinal permeability, release of bacterial endotoxin, creation of carcinogenic secondary bile salts/polycyclic aromatic hydrocarbons/N-nitroso compounds/heterocyclic aromatic amines, and vascular disease-fueling TMAO. Yes, it is easier for our body to digest and process meat. We don't rely on our microbiome as much for that. So you may not feel any discomfort, but keep in mind what's happening inside you. Silent but deadly.

So how do we break this vicious cycle? It starts with a carb intervention. But let's address the hurdles we need to clear before we can begin the program.

Constipation?

First and foremost, if you're dealing with gas and bloating we absolutely need to make sure there's no constipation. This is by far the number one cause of gas and bloating that I see in my clinic. It has its own vicious cycle—methane gas slows gut motility, causing constipation. Then, constipation increases the amount of gas we produce from our food. In other words, gas causes constipation, which causes more gas. I've found in my practice that if my patients maintain bowel regularity and correct the constipation, they feel so much better and the gas and bloating issues go away. But first you have to know whether or not constipation is present, and the truth is that it's more common than most people realize.

Even if you don't *feel* constipated, your ears should be perking up if you have a history of constipation, ever strain to poop, drop little nuggets or turds, or sometimes go a day without a movement. And here's the crazy thing . . . even if you have diarrhea, believe it or not you may be constipated. The most severe constipation presents with diarrhea. Basically what happens is you have a column of impacted stool stuck somewhere in your colon, and the solid stuff piles up behind the "log jam" but the liquid can still sneak through the cracks and crevices to come down to the bottom and come out loose. It's very confusing to both the doctor and the patient because severe constipation is manifesting with loose bowel movements. We call this overflow diarrhea, and the treatment is actually to purge the colon to relieve the blockage. So if there's any change in your bowel habits or a possibility of constipation, you should ask your primary care doctor to check an abdominal x-ray to rule out constipation or (under the guidance of your doctor) drink a bottle of magnesium citrate to initiate a colon purge and essentially have a fresh start.

You absolutely will not have success on a plant-based diet if you are trying to ramp up fiber consumption while being constipated. In my clinic, we don't even consider dietary changes until the constipation is corrected. I'd recommend consulting with your primary care doctor or a gastroenterologist locally to get the constipation under control before moving forward with a dietary overhaul.

Food sensitivity versus food allergy

The next thing we need to understand is whether you may be experiencing a food sensitivity or a food allergy. I hear a lot of people describing their gas and bloating as a food allergy. To me, this is more than just semantics. If you have a specific food that you're proven to be allergic to, then you actually do have a medical reason to eliminate that food. Although it is technically possible to build tolerance to a food allergy, it is a fragile, complex process that needs to be done under physician supervision. Most will just eliminate the food. Why? Because a food allergy is your immune system reacting when it's stimulated by that particular food. The most common food allergies are to milk, fish, shellfish, eggs, nuts and peanuts, wheat, and soy. When people with an allergy eat these foods the immune system goes on the attack, launching IgE (Immunoglobulin E) antibodies like missiles to attack the allergen. This process releases chemicals that cause an allergic reaction, which can include itchiness, hives, swollen lips, a throat that closes up, trouble breathing, or even loss of consciousness. This is very different from a food sensitivity, where you may feel bloating, gas, diarrhea, abdominal discomfort, and fatigue. It's an important distinction because if you really do have a food allergy, then you absolutely should eliminate that food from your diet. But if it's a food sensitivity, then it's not your immune system reacting and you should be able to train your gut to be able to process it. If there's any question whatsoever, you need to work with your doctor to determine whether or not it's a food allergy. There's no one test that is adequately reliable to answer this question alone, and therefore you need the assistance of a qualified health professional.

Gluten

Let's deal with gluten for the last time. There are three major groups of people who should not be consuming gluten, and there are two groups who should be consuming gluten. Everyone falls into one of these five groups. For what it's worth, the latter two groups make up at least 90 percent of the American population. I'm going to describe each one and walk you through how you can determine whether or not you meet these criteria.

You *should not consume gluten* if you have:

CELIAC DISEASE—If you have celiac disease, you need to be 100 percent gluten-free for the rest of your life. Continued gluten consumption isn't just disruptive, it's dangerous and can lead to small bowel T-cell lymphoma, which is almost universally fatal. About 1 percent of Americans have celiac disease. Classic symptoms of celiac disease include diarrhea, bloating, gas, abdominal pain, and weight loss. Occasionally you'll find it in someone who is constipated. I also think of celiac anytime I see someone with low iron levels. The intestinal damage from celiac affects the small intestine, where iron is typically absorbed. If you have any of these symptoms or are worried that you may have celiac disease, there are two tests for you to consider that can definitively tell you whether or not you have celiac:

Genetic testing for HLA-DQ2 or DQ8: In order to have celiac you must meet three criteria—have the genes, consume gluten, and activate the gene through dysbiosis. In other words, it's impossible to have celiac disease if you don't have the gene. So you can have your blood analyzed for the celiac genes, and if they're not present, you don't have celiac. If you do have the gene, it doesn't necessarily mean you have or will ever have celiac disease. In fact, there's a 97 percent chance that you don't have celiac despite having the gene. But if you are genetically positive, it means that celiac is possible and therefore additional testing is necessary to determine whether or not it's present.

Upper endoscopy with biopsies of the small intestine: This is the gold standard test for determining whether or not celiac is present. Basically, you will need to see a gastroenterologist such as myself to be scheduled for this procedure. After you are sedated, a doctor will run a flexible tube the size of a pinkie (a cute pinkie! Not too big!) with a light and camera down into your stomach and small intestine. This allows biopsies to be taken from the small intestine—two from the first segment of the duodenum and four from the second segment. The entire procedure typically takes just five minutes. It's important for you to consume gluten in the days leading up to the procedure because that's the only way to tell if gluten is causing damage to the intestine. It is these biopsies that ultimately tell the story. A pathologist uses special criteria for evaluating for celiac disease called the Marsh classification to determine what damage, if any, is present. Marsh grade can be from I to IV, with IV being the most severe. Traditionally, grade III or IV disease is classified as celiac. But this is a spectrum, and in recent years there have been studies showing that Grades I and II are celiac, too. The reason I'm breaking this down for you is to tell you that blood tests for celiac disease are usually positive for Grade III or IV disease yet usually negative for Grade I or II. So the blood test can be negative and be wrong! Therefore, if you suspect you have celiac, you should skip the blood test and do either the genetic test or move forward with upper endoscopy with biopsies. The vast majority of celiac disease that I diagnose is Marsh I, and these people do incredibly well when I put them on a gluten-free diet. But I would have missed them if I'd just done the traditional blood test.

WHEAT ALLERGY: This isn't necessarily a reaction to gluten, but it is a reaction to proteins found in wheat. Similar to other food allergies, the results are generally dramatic: hives, lip or throat swelling, difficulty breathing, or anaphylaxis. GI symptoms such as diarrhea and abdominal pain may also be present. Wheat allergy almost always develops in childhood, and affects 0.4 percent of American kids. It is extremely rare to develop wheat allergy as an adult unless you have occupational exposure, so bear that in mind. If you have wheat allergy, that would also be grounds to be completely wheat-free. Since it may not be gluten, it's possible that barley and rye can remain on your menu. Testing for a wheat allergy is not quite as straightforward and decisive as it is for celiac disease, so it's best to address this issue with a qualified health professional. That said, if you're having hives, lip or throat swelling, difficulty breathing, or anaphylaxis in relation to *any* food, I'd recommend you stop eating that food. Pretty straightforward.

NON-CELIAC GLUTEN SENSITIVITY WITH EXTRAINTESTINAL SYMPTOMS: Okay, of the five categories that I'm going to describe, this is the one that we're working the hardest to figure out. The challenge is that we use one diagnosis to describe a whole bunch of different conditions, all of which are exceedingly rare. It's incredibly difficult to study a heterogenous group of extremely rare conditions. They are even rarer than celiac disease. These conditions can occur outside the intestine, may be tied back to gluten, and may improve on a gluten-free diet. Specific symptoms I'm referring to are joint or muscle pain, leg or arm numbness, or neurologic symptoms like altered mental status, loss of balance or muscle control, or a rash. The classic rash is called dermatitis herpetiformis and is characterized by an itchy, vesicular rash symmetrically on the elbows, knees, butt, and trunk. Psoriasis can also be associated with celiac disease. If you or your doctor suspect celiac, it's absolutely imperative that you have celiac testing done. For example, 85 percent of adults with dermatitis herpetiformis actually have celiac. Similarly, antibodies to gluten are found in 85 percent of people with gluten-related neurologic conditions, often in association with

Marsh I histology on small intestine biopsies. If you definitively test negative for celiac disease yet wonder if gluten is causing your arthritis, leg or arm numbness, neurologic symptoms, or rash, then it would make sense to try a gluten-free diet for a few months to assess your response. If you improve, you can challenge yourself by reintroducing gluten and if symptoms come back, then you have your answer. Of course, this would be done under the guidance of a qualified health professional.

You *should consume gluten* if you are:

COMPLETELY SYMPTOM FREE: Let me keep this short and sweet. If you have absolutely no symptoms and absolutely no reason to suspect you have celiac disease or any of these conditions, you should *not* be on a gluten-free diet. As we discussed in Chapter 4, you are unintentionally damaging your gut and increasing your risk for other conditions like coronary artery disease. 'Nuff said!

NON-CELIAC GLUTEN SENSITIVITY WITH ONLY DIGESTIVE SYMPTOMS: If you suffer exclusively from digestive symptoms after ingestion of gluten-containing foods—bloating, gas, distension, abdominal pain, diarrhea, or constipation—then you absolutely need to have testing to rule out celiac disease. But if those tests prove decisively that you do not have it, then we need to regroup.

Recent research reveals that for many people, gluten may not be the real culprit. Consider a study in which researchers gave people with "gluten sensitivity" an oatmeal bar every day for a week. Concealed within the bar was one of three things: a placebo (sugar), gluten, or fructans. Fructans are short-chain carbohydrates that you'll find in gluten-containing foods (wheat, barley, and rye). Every person was exposed to a different bar after taking a break for a week to let his or her system settle down. During each week they measured the average GI symptom scores for each person. Here's what they found: Compared to placebo, the patients actually had *fewer* GI symptoms during the week that they were eating the gluten bar. Fewer symptoms! Let that register for a moment. Then when they ate the fructan bar they saw a big increase in digestive symptoms relative to both the placebo and the gluten bar. In other words, most people who have non-celiac gluten sensitivity aren't even sensitive to gluten. They're sensitive to fructans. And their symptoms are being triggered because they have underlying dysbiosis with irritable bowel syndrome. So what are these fructans? We will cover them in the next section.

How to be gluten-free and still nurture your gut

So what's a sensible approach to gluten consumption? Well if you absolutely *need* to be gluten-free, then I would recommend paying special attention to your whole-grain intake. Since wheat is the dominant form of whole grain in the United States, you need to make sure that you're adequately supporting your gut microbiome. Thankfully, there are some delicious gluten-free whole grains available for you to routinely consume: quinoa, buckwheat, millet, sorghum, oats, and brown rice. Get them into your belly! On the flip side, if gluten is a part of your diet, which it should be for most of you, I'm not encouraging you to go eat more processed foods. Most gluten-containing foods are processed foods. What I encourage you to eat is more unprocessed or minimally processed wheat, barley, and rye. Look for whole-grain products, like whole-grain bread and pasta when they are called for. But remember not to overdo it. Moderation is just fine.

Let's talk about FODMAPs

Just a few pages ago we were chatting about how the gut microbiome has shown the ability to adapt to lactose exposure. We also talked about the Hadzas' seasonal variation in diet and how when they ate more berries they trained their microbiome to process fructans. Then we discovered that most people with GI symptoms from gluten don't actually have a problem with gluten, but likely have underlying irritable bowel syndrome being triggered by—here's that word again—fructans. So what are we referring to here? We're talking about FODMAPs. Perhaps you've heard this term dropped in conversation. FODMAPs are simple or short-chain carbohydrates found in our plant food. FODMAP is actually an acronym—fermentable oligosaccharides, disaccharides, monosaccharides, and polyols. You need to memorize that because I'm going to test you on it later. Just kidding—no, I'm not.

Anyway, these FODMAPs are foods that are, by definition, fermentable. They're also poorly absorbed, which means that they draw water into the intestine and can cause diarrhea. By escaping digestion, they reach the lower intestine where the gut bacteria reside. These gut bacteria then feast on these carbs, in the process producing hydrogen gas along with potentially other by-products. We rely on our gut microbiota to work their magic and process these foods for us with their glycoside hydrolase enzymes. In people who have damage to their microbiota, such as those with irritable bowel syndrome, the loss of digestive capacity can lead to maldigestion, gas, bloating, discomfort, and diarrhea.

There are five categories of FODMAPs to be aware of. As you're reading this section, if you suffer from food sensitivity, consider the foods within a specific category. Do you have a sensitivity to more than one?

Lactose—A disaccharide found in dairy products like milk, ice cream, and some cheeses. For aforementioned reasons, I support the elimination of lactose from the diet. Many of you will see improvement in digestive symptoms with this simple move.

Fructose—A simple sugar found in many fruits (cherries, watermelon, apples), some veggies (asparagus, Jerusalem artichokes), high-fructose corn syrup, and honey.

Fructans—Oligosaccharides found in a variety of foods, including gluten-containing grains (wheat, barley, rye) as well as fruits and veggies (garlic, onions).

Galacto-oligosaccharides (GOS)—Complex sugars classically found in beans. *Toot toot!*

Polyols—Sugar alcohols like mannitol and sorbitol, often found in artificial sweeteners and some fruits and veggies.

Since FODMAPs can cause digestive symptoms, we should eliminate them, right? Not so fast, my friend! We need to be careful about vilifying these parts of our food when in fact they can be incredibly healthy for us. For example, fructans and galacto-oligosaccharides are prebiotics! As discussed in Chapter 3, this means that they are fuel to grow and energize the healthy bacteria in your gut and ultimately yield more postbiotic SCFAs.

Perhaps you've heard of the low FODMAP diet? The idea is that appropriate restriction of FODMAPs can reduce digestive distress in people with irritable bowel syndrome. And for some patients with irritable bowel syndrome this does work. The problem is that many people, doctors included, have misinterpreted these studies to mean that FODMAPs should be eliminated permanently. But this cuts against the Golden Rule. Plant-based diversity is the greatest predictor of a healthy gut. And, again, FODMAPs are actually incredibly healthy and most of them are prebiotics.

So what happens if we permanently restrict FODMAPs? Their restriction, in the setting of the low FODMAP diet, may lead to harm of the beneficial bacteria and a drop in total bacterial count. So now we have fewer SCFA-producing bacteria and simultaneously are restricting prebiotics. This is a recipe for less postbiotic SCFAs. Not good.

Finally, the restrictive nature of the low FODMAP diet can lead to micronutrient deficiencies. In one study the low FODMAP diet led to significant declines in several important micronutrients: retinol, thiamin, riboflavin, and calcium. What this means is that if we want a healthy gut, then we actually need our fructans and galacto-oligosaccharides.

It's important to recognize that the low FODMAP diet, as developed at Monash University in Australia, was never meant to be a permanent elimination diet. Instead, it was meant to be a temporary FODMAP restriction for two to six weeks followed by a systematic reintroduction of the FODMAPs. The actual point of the diet is that our food sensitivities may vary among the categories of FODMAPs and that increased awareness of this can make us smart consumers. This is exactly how these FODMAP categories should be used: If you have difficulty in dealing with one particular category, then you know where the weakness in your gut lies and that you may need to go slow and easy on building up strength there. If you want a list of foods that fall into certain FODMAP categories, email me at fodmap@theplantfedgut .com and I'll send you what you need.

Bringing it back full circle now, we know that following the Golden Rule and maximizing plant-based diversity in our diet is the key to a healthier gut. It offers the prebiotic fiber and micronutrients in both balance and variety. This is fiber fuel for health. The result is a strong gut microbiota that's firing on all cylinders and optimizing health throughout our entire body.

But many of us are going to have difficulty in processing our plant carbohydrates, specifically fiber and FODMAPs. The reason for this is that we humans rely almost entirely on our gut microbiota to do this work for us, so if the gut is damaged, then the struggle is real!

It's incredibly important to understand that the plant foods we need the most to get our gut stronger are also the same foods that cause digestive distress in people with a damaged gut. Yes, it's frustrating. But it's the way it works, and we're about results so it's important to know the rules of the game. So how do we break this vicious cycle, get our guts back, and start enjoying more plant food in our diet? We have to treat our gut like a muscle and train it. Think of Rocky, running through the streets of Philadelphia and up the steps of the Museum of Art. He didn't just wake up one morning and do that. It took time and effort to build up that level of fitness to propel him to the championship. That's what the Fiber Fueled 4 Weeks (see Chapter 10) is going to be for you. It's a structured four-week plan to start from scratch and build that gut.

Ultimately, the plan will help you understand the FODMAPs your gut is good with and which ones it needs help with. As we progressively introduce fiber and FODMAPs, it's important to start low and go slow. This may be the most important sentence in the chapter, so please sear this one into your brain. To properly train our gut, we need to start low and go slow with fiber and FODMAPs. Low and slow to grow—that's the motto. You feel me? That's the "Rocky" approach to building up your gut fitness. You can do this. And I'm here to help you.

To view the 25+ scientific references cited in this chapter, please visit me online at www.theplantfedgut.com/research/.

6

Fermentation Nation Rising

The benefits of fermented foods for gut health and where to start

*A*re you ready to unlock the full nutritional value of your food and take your plant-based diversity to a level that you didn't even know existed? Allow me to introduce you to one of my secret weapons—fermented foods.

I'm obsessed with fermented foods. They are really cool because they give our food a complete makeover on several levels. You start with something already delicious, sprinkle some fermentation magic (or science) on top, and the ingredient is transformed into a new healthy food.

At the crossroads of our gut microbiota and food lies fermentation. What happens inside a jar of fermenting sauerkraut is a microcosm of what's happening inside our guts. It's the same process and the same concept but it's happening before our eyes on our kitchen counters: millions of invisible microbes, working in a coordinated symphony right there in front of us. We can't see them, but we can see and taste the difference in their work. It's quite remarkable.

Every single culture in human history has fermented foods as a celebrated part of their food tradition. You have sauerkraut from Germany, kvass from Russia, kimchi from Korea, natto and miso from Japan, tempeh from Indonesia, and if you've ever had Ethiopian food you know that spongy tangy fermented bread called injera. Even sourdough bread, made by fermenting flour, has roots in the California and Klondike Gold Rush—that's what those guys in the mountains used to eat. If you study the food traditions of any culture, you will find fermentation at its heart. Sadly, we let go of our traditional foods in exchange for hypersterile, chemical-laden convenience foods offered up by our food industry. But it's time to say, "Enough!" Today we can embrace fermented foods as the next frontier in our quest for plant-based diversity. A little fermented food every day goes a long way.

My introduction to fermented foods

As a kid, I never would have dreamed that fermented foods would be a future obsession. But the more I learned about SCFAs, gut microbiota, and the power of plants for gut health, the more curious I became about fermentation. So it was serendipity that one of my patients came in raving about how helpful sauerkraut and pickles had been for his digestive issues. That was it—I couldn't wait another day. I had to try it.

So I set out to make my first batch of sauerkraut. I found the recipe and the process to be so refreshingly basic. It's just water, salt, and cabbage. That's it. So simple. No need to add any starter culture—all the microbes you need are already part of the cabbage microbiome. But sinking my hands into the chopped cabbage and working on it to release some of the juices and soften it made me feel connected to the food. It was a living food.

I popped my mason jar of water, salt, and cabbage on the kitchen counter where it sat for weeks. Yes, weeks! My wife and I were a little

FERMENTATION NATION RISING **119**

bit scared of it, to be honest. It felt so weird to have food that's not in the fridge. How could this be okay to eat?

After a few weeks, we tried it. It was . . . very crunchy! I didn't expect that. It was tangy and acidic, too—and delicious. I took more bites. Many more. I was in fermented nirvana. It's been a daily part of my life ever since.

The bacterial artistry behind fermentation and healthy soil

Perhaps you haven't spent a lot of time thinking about food decomposition, but this is exactly what Louis Pasteur was thinking about when he discovered modern germ theory in the 1860s. By studying how wine is created from grapes and how milk spoils, he started to understand that microorganisms are at the heart of all of it. Understanding the process of food decomposition is an important part of assessing the nutritional value of our food.

These bacteria that are responsible for the decomposition of our perishable items—aren't they a bad thing? Certainly they frustrate and enrage us when we miss that preciously small window of avocado perfection, or when we find some lettuce we forgot in the back of our fridge that now seems like some sort of nightmare science experiment. So, yes, when our food becomes inedible it's kind of a drag, but really that's nature saying, "Hey, you had your chance to eat this food, now I'm taking it back."

It doesn't just take it back, though—when we compost our food, we're actually empowering nature to do its thing and recycle it: Similar to digestion, the microbes work in teams and use varied enzymes to break down and transform our food. Allowing the natural life cycle of dead plant matter to unfold produces humic substances—humic acids, fulvic acids, and humin. These humic substances form the basis of healthy soil, and healthy soil grows healthy plants, which feed our microbiota to help us be healthy humans. It's a beautiful part of the circle of life.

Soil health is vastly underrated and something we should take very seriously for the health of both ourselves and our planet. Bottom line: Your food is only as healthy as your soil, which means that you are only as healthy as your soil. We desperately need microbe- and humic-enriched soil. But yes, along that path of transformation to humus what starts as food does eventually become inedible. We don't need to fear this; we simply need to accept that the life cycle of our food has passed the window of human nutrition and is now moving toward soil nutrition.

But here's where the magic comes in: Microbes cause degradation, but when you tweak those microbes you can transform the process dramatically. That's fermentation in a nutshell. Instead of allowing a food to decompose and break down, you introduce a different band of bacteria that will actually prolong the life of the food and alter it. We do this with the bacteria that naturally live on the plant. They're already there as a part of the plant's microbiome; all you have to do is create the right conditions to be successful.

Let's take sauerkraut as an example. The first thing that happens when you make sauerkraut by fermenting cabbage is that anaerobic bacteria begin producing healthy acids to drop the pH of the solution. Anaerobic means they thrive where there is no oxygen, so by putting the cabbage underwater you're creating the proper conditions for anaerobes to grow. As this happens, the acid levels become too high for many bacteria, allowing *Leuconostoc mesenteroides* to take over within twenty-four hours, producing more healthy acids to drop the pH even further. If you're making sauerkraut at home, you'll know *Leuconostoc* is present when you start seeing the bubbles form. Over the following week, the environment becomes increasingly acidic, which leads to the growth of *Lactobacillus plantarum*, the primary bacteria responsible for transforming saltwater cabbage into kraut.

Back in Chapter 3 we discussed how SCFAs (short-chain fatty acids) actually reduce the pH in the colon, which inhibits pathogenic bacteria and promotes the growth of SCFA-producing commensal bacteria. You can apply that same concept here to our ferment—the drop in pH inhibits pathogenic as well as decomposing species and promotes the growth of the right species responsible for fermentation. This is the first example of how the process in a mason jar can mimic what's happening in our gut. Isn't it amazing that by altering the blend of bacteria, we can actually inhibit food spoilage and prolong the life of our food?

How microbes clean up our mess and don't even get a "thank you"

As a demonstration of the cleansing, restoring power of microbes in nature, consider the Deepwater Horizon oil spill in 2010. This oil spill dumped an estimated 4.2 million barrels of oil in the Gulf of Mexico. Folks, that's more than a billion venti Starbucks filled with oil and dumped into the ocean. To me, dumping even one venti Starbucks' worth of oil would be a disgrace. It was an environmental catastrophe, causing widespread harm to marine life and its ecosystems from the ocean floor to the surface, extending from deep water to the coastal tidal marshes. It was the largest offshore oil spill in U.S. history, and frankly it was disgusting. But we're not seeing oil in the Gulf water or beaches anymore. So how did the ocean heal itself?

A group of researchers from the Lawrence Berkeley National Laboratory recently showed that bacterial species survived within the oil plumes and together in cooperative fashion, these bacteria took up the challenge of degrading 4.2 million barrels. The study discovered that it was the right bacteria working at the right time in a cooperative fashion to clean the ocean. Personally, I think we need to stop destroying this planet and hoping our friendly Earthly microbes will bail us out, but to witness the incredible healing power of these microbes in real time is amazing, isn't it? This concept of bacteria functioning in teams with the right microbe stepping up at the right time is the same process you'll find in fermentation, healthy soil production, and even carbohydrate digestion in your gut. Invisible microbes are everywhere, doing amazing things without us even recognizing them.

A brief history of fermentation and food preservation

Fermented foods are at the heart of our human origin story. Our ancestors had a major problem that they needed to overcome: They had no way of preserving food. It held back the growth of the tribe, required constant attention to food finding, and forced the nomadic lifestyle on them. There was no settling down. For human civilization to move forward—organized society, cities, an economy, all of it—we needed to leave the famine behind and find food security by stockpiling and delayed-return subsistence. Once again, the microbes came to our rescue.

We don't know exactly when fermentation was discovered. Fourteen-thousand-year-old bread was recently found at a Natufian hunter-gatherer camp in Jordan. There's a cave in Israel where they found a wheat/barley-based beer mixture dating back thirteen thousand years. In Sweden there are ninety-two-hundred-year-old pits in the ground used to preserve large quantities of fish. In China researchers found a nine-thousand-year-old rice, honey, and fruit libation similar to rice wine. The bottom line is that fermentation started popping up in cultures around the world at a similar time, and appears to be one of the major developments contributing to the rise of human civilization.

For thousands of years this was one of our principle forms of food preservation and a celebrated part of our ancient traditions. But in the nineteenth and twentieth centuries we developed new approaches to food preservation: canning, pasteurization, numerous preservatives, refrigeration, and freezing. Our dependence on fermentation for preservation was marginalized and, particularly in a melting-pot nation such as the United States, food traditions that included fermented foods were lost. Did we make a major mistake by turning to new forms of food preservation? I'd say so.

All food preservation techniques work by altering the microbes. For example, canning works through sterilization. Food is heated to destroy the bacteria, then sealed in a vacuum-tight container. The sealed, sterile contents aren't exposed to microbes and their enzymes of food decomposition and therefore remain preserved until the can is opened. But is this completely benign? We previously learned that an apple has one hundred million microbes in its microbiome, many of which are known to be beneficial to humans. To sterilize is to destroy the plant microbiome and any health benefits that would come from it.

How about the thousands of chemical preservatives in our processed foods? Consider the turkey or ham that sits in a deli refrigerator for months on end, with a few slices taken off every once in a while. The bread that stays soft for weeks without hardening or molding. The crackers wrapped up in a box that are as fresh as the day they were manufactured. Since processed foods are part of our daily world, we don't spend enough time questioning them or considering how unnatural they are.

I think you know where I'm going here. To pasteurize is to transiently kill the microbes and sterilize our food. But most of our food today is on a whole new level—not just sterilized, but actually crossbred with chemical preservatives that are developed with the intention of inhibiting microbes and their food-processing enzymes.

Our Food and Drug Administration labels them as "benign" or "nontoxic" to the consumer. I can't help but consider what these chemicals designed to retard microbes do when introduced to the dense population of microbes in our colon. In one study, sulfites damaged these four probiotic superstars: *Lactobacillus casei, L. plantarum, L.*

rhamnosus, and *Streptococcus thermophilus*. Those were the only four tested, so we don't know what happens with the others. There's certainly room for more research to help us understand the best way to preserve our food without compromising our gut microbiota. In the meantime, I'll happily munch my organic fruits and veggies.

Unleash the full potential in your food

Food preservation doesn't always have to be about destroying the microbes. Fermentation is one of the rare examples of food processing that actually makes our food even *more* healthy. When you think of fermentation, think of transformation. The taste and appearance get a reboot. We're breeding new microbes, transforming fiber, and generating bioactive peptides and polyphenols. All parts of our food have the possibility of changing. It's absolutely fascinating stuff that the scientific community is just beginning to understand.

You've noticed that fermented foods are often sour to some degree? As we discussed with sauerkraut, fermentation causes the release of acids that lower the pH and alter the balance of bacteria. These acids often have health-promoting properties themselves beyond just altering the balance of bacteria. For example, lactic acid has been shown to reduce inflammation and have antioxidant properties in the gut. Therefore, if a fraction of the lactic acid found in a ferment makes it to the small intestine, benefits ensue. Studies have shown that vinegar, the product of fermentation of alcohol, can improve insulin sensitivity, improve fullness after meals to promote weight loss, and may lower blood pressure and cholesterol.

The acidic environment helps to grow the right microbes. Fermented foods with live active cultures can contain upward of a billion microorganisms per gram or milliliter of food. Compared to the hyper-sterilized diet in the Western world, the consumption of fermented foods could increase the number of microbes in the diet by up to 10,000 fold. In the study comparing five days on a plant-based versus animal-based diet, Drs. Lawrence David and Peter Turnbaugh were surprised to find that foodborne microbes survived transit and were metabolically active, suggesting that the microbes naturally occurring in and on our food really may provide benefit to humans.

But before these microbes begin their incredible journey through our intestines, they first get to work on unpacking the hidden nutrition in our food. Working in teams, they use their enzymes like the tools of a mechanic. For example, *Lactobacillus* species have specific enzymes—glycoside hydrolases, esterases, decarboxylases, and phenolic acid reductases—to enhance conversion of health-promoting flavonoids in cherries and broccoli into biologically active metabolites. These are the same *Lactobacillus* species that grow in your gut when you consume prebiotic fiber. We talked before about how glycoside hydrolases are the enzymes used to break down fiber, and here you see them showing up in our fermented food, the point being that what the microbes do during fermentation mirrors what they do during digestion.

Microbial enzymes can be natural pharmaceuticals

Nattokinase is an enzyme produced when boiled soybeans are fermented to form natto, a traditional food in Japan. Natto has been used as a folk remedy for diseases of the heart and blood vessels for hundreds of years, and now we know why. Recent research has found that nattokinase has potent clot-busting, blood pressure–lowering, cholesterol-controlling, platelet-stunning, and plaque-stabilizing properties. Basically it's like taking aspirin, heparin, blood pressure pills, and a statin all in one. The perfect cardiac cocktail. It comes as no surprise that drug companies are trying to figure out how they can turn this into a pill. But I say, why don't we just eat natto?

These enzymes allow our microbes to create nutrition where it didn't previously exist. For example, these microbial magicians are able to synthesize vitamin K and B vitamins—folate, riboflavin, and B_{12}—from non-vitamin precursors. Melatonin and GABA are both synthesized, too. Melatonin is a powerful antioxidant that I've seen help people with acid reflux. GABA has a calming effect on the brain and helps regulate blood pressure.

Any part of the food can be transformed during fermentation. For example, the microbes create supercharged forms of fiber called exopolysaccharides. They've been shown to inhibit unhealthy microbes, regulate the immune system, squash inflammation, lower cholesterol, and even protect against cancer. If that sounds an awful lot like what prebiotic fiber and SCFAs were shown to do in Chapter 3, that's because that's exactly what's happening—prebiotic exopolysaccharides produced during fermentation are then fermented by intestinal microbiota to release postbiotic SCFAs. The point being, our gut thrives on diversity of fiber and, by creating exopolysaccharides, we are adding to that diversity to support our gut microbiome. Powerful stuff, folks.

We're only beginning to study fermented foods and the bioactive molecules the microbes create. The proteins, phytochemicals, and polyphenols in food may all undergo transformation during fermentation. Here are just a few examples of what we are learning:

- Fermentation of red ginseng increases the number of bioactive saponins and helps to control blood sugar.
- Twenty-five different antioxidant peptides have been found in different types of sourdough.
- Fermentation of soy milk with *Lactobacillus paracasei* or *L. plantarum* activates isoflavones to increase bone volume and thickness in the fight against osteoporosis.

Fermentation can also practice addition by subtraction, meaning that it can enhance the nutritive qualities in the food by reducing the anti-nutritional compounds. Specifically, fermentation is known to reduce gluten, phytic acid content, and FODMAPs. For this reason, people with IBS generally tolerate sourdough bread better than traditional wheat bread. Oh, and those vicious, life-threatening lectins you've been hearing about? Fermentation removes 95 percent of them.

Just like bacteria can help us clean up an oil spill, they can also help us biodegrade and reduce pesticide residues on our plants. You can probably predict what I'm about to say, because there's a theme that keeps reemerging in nature. Teams of microbes have hydrolytic enzymes that allow them to dismantle and deactivate the pesticides.

FAQ

So if fermented foods are so great, what's stopping us? Let me take a few of the concerns head on.

Is it safe to eat fermented foods?

As long as fermentation is properly done, fermented foods are absolutely safe. This isn't creating unhealthy, contaminated food, it is actually cleaning it up. People worry about getting a bad bug or gastroenteritis, yet there are literally no reported cases of food poisoning. The large outbreaks of *Salmonella* or *E. coli* you've heard about are related to contamination of raw vegetables. Understand two things about these outbreaks: First, the process of fermentation would eliminate these pathogenic bacteria. Remember, that's why wine was added to water in ancient times. But second and even more important, these are the consequences of industrial animal agriculture. There is no great way to dispose of the feces, and ultimately the large ponds of stool run off when it rains.

What about botulism?

Botulism is a rare but very serious neurological disease caused by a bacteria called *Clostridium botulinum*. People often inappropriately associate it with fermentation because they know that botulism can be the result of food preservation gone wrong. But to be clear, botulism is associated with canning, not fermentation. *C. botulinum* can produce a spore that's resistant to high temperature, surviving the pasteurization step in canning and then thriving in the oxygen-deprived environment of the can.

On the flip side, fermentation intentionally avoids high heat (which would kill the bacteria, including the good ones) and instead allows those friendly microbes to produce acid, which destroys *C. botulinum.*

How will I know that I'm doing it properly and growing the right bacteria?

It's actually rather simple. Just use your senses and be smart and intuitive as you observe the process. Do you see something that looks like mold—fuzzy and round, potentially colored blue, black, or pink, generally on the surface of the ferment? Technically you can skim it off, but I tend to err on the side of just starting over. I also start over if there's anything that smells off or looks funny in the ferment. Point being, I play it safe.

Can fermented foods cause cancer?

If we're discussing all fermented foods, then yes, processed meat or fish have been associated with colorectal, nasopharyngeal, esophageal, lung, stomach, and pancreatic cancer. When it comes to fermented veggies, the main concern has been stomach cancer. Epidemiologic studies from East Asia have found an association between stomach cancer and pickled vegetable consumption. Stomach cancer is a huge problem in East Asia, where it is the second most common cancer.

Most cases are the result of *Helicobacter pylori*, a carcinogenic bacteria that lives in the stomach of 60 to 70 percent of Japanese and Koreans. Still, only a fraction of colonized individuals develop stomach cancer. So where do fermented veggies fit in? It turns out that salt and its by-products actually accelerate the inflammation and cancer development in the stomach lining. Should we be concerned and avoid fermented veggies with salt? No. We should moderate our salt intake, which is a smart move from the get-go. We should also recognize that these foods are consumed at every meal in East Asia, and that we're going to be consuming them at a fraction of the quantity. We also have a much lower prevalence of *H. pylori* in the United States, and most strains are not the one widely associated with cancer.

Two main points here: First, consuming anything to ridiculous excess is bad for you. We need oxygen to live, but pure oxygen is actually toxic. Second, let's all just take a deep breath, partially to just chill for a moment; partially to reinforce the point that oxygen is completely safe at a normal dose, even if we know it can be dangerous if you have too much of it, too. There can always be too much of a good thing.

Fermented favorites

Now that we've addressed some of the big themes in fermented foods, let me introduce you to some of the superstars of fermentation:

Sauerkraut

Where would you place cabbage on a list of the world's healthiest foods? Is it top ten? Even top five? We already know that cabbage is incredibly good for us—low in calories, high in nutrients like vitamin C, high in prebiotic fiber to support a healthy gut and unleash SCFAs throughout the body. Cabbage is a part of the cruciferous family, like broccoli, cauliflower, Brussels sprouts, and kale. That's an all-star list, in part because cruciferous veggies contain glucosinolates, which are potent cancer-fighting phytochemicals. The problem is that glucosinolates need to be converted into their active form as isothiocyanates in order to fight cancer. In 2002, a group of Finnish researchers showed that fermenting cabbage produces the enzymes necessary to unleash these isothiocyanates. It's a powerful example of fermentation amping up an already healthy food and taking it to another level.

Make your own sauerkraut!

It's fun, delicious, and healthy! Before you get started, let me just say that part of making fermented foods is experimenting and trying new things. Rather than searching the Internet for specific proportions, I'd really encourage you to pull an Emeril and just go *BAM* and throw some stuff in the mason jar and see what happens. It's more fun. Here's how you do it:

1. Lightly rinse your cabbage. Nothing aggressive that would kill the bacteria. Peel back the top two layers of leaves.
2. Chop the cabbage to your desired kraut thickness. I like it thick! Put your hands into the cabbage and work on it to break it up and soften. Feel that connection to the food.
3. Pack into a 1-quart mason jar. Feel free to add garlic cloves, caraway seeds, or spices if you like. No recipes here! It's fun to experiment. I use a wooden sauerkraut pounder to pack it in. Fill the jar about 75 percent.
4. Add a fermentation weight on top. There are glass fermentation weights available commercially. Some people clean a rock from their yard and others use a few cabbage leaves for packing. The key is to use something heavy enough to keep everything submerged.
5. Make a sea salt brine by mixing 1 cup of water with roughly 1¼ teaspoons of sea salt. I honestly don't measure, I just go by taste. It should taste salty, but not so salty that you

wouldn't take a sip of it. The water needs to be chlorine free, so either use distilled water, or boil water and let it return to room temperature. The salt needs to be iodine free, which is why I use sea salt.

6. Pour the sea salt brine over the chopped cabbage and cover with the fermentation weight. You want to completely cover the cabbage and weight but still leave a little room at the top. I remove any bits and pieces of cabbage that float to the surface.

7. Cover the mason jar, ideally with an airlock that allows it to vacuum seal and burp on its own. If you don't use a valve to allow gas to escape, you'll need to "burp" the kraut once a day to release pressure from the gas that builds up.

8. Place in a cool location for 1 to 4 weeks to ferment. Ideal temperature is less than 70 degrees Fahrenheit. I usually start tasting after about a week and find that it gets better with age.

9. If you notice a white, powdery yeast at the surface, that's kahm yeast. It's common, it's not mold, and it's not harmful to your health. Simply scoop it off the surface with a paper towel. If it's fuzzy looking, blue, or green, and looks like mold, that's because it is. Some people remove it and still eat the ferment. I personally toss the batch and start over.

10. Two things that have a big effect on fermentation are the storage temperature and salinity of the brine. The cooler the temperature, the slower the ferment progresses, which is usually a good thing. Too fast and it can cause mold. In similar fashion, increased salinity also slows down the process and protects against mold.

If at any point you decide that you want to stop progression of the fermentation, just throw it in the fridge. It's like shouting "Freeze!" to the microbes. Fermentation pauses and the kraut is good for months stored there.

Kimchi

There's not much separating kimchi from sauerkraut; they're really just two celebrated expressions of fermented cabbage from cultures on opposite sides of the world. In the case of kimchi, it is often mixed with other vegetables such as onions, garlic, hot peppers, and radishes to generate a spicy fermented salad of sorts. Once again, microbes are the stars here, and in the process of transforming, kimchi rewards us with phytochemicals, healthy acids, volatile compounds, and free amino acids.

Kimchi is a celebrated tradition in Korea, and each region has its own unique spin on the dish. It's normal to have a small side of kimchi with nearly every meal, and the average Korean eats forty-eight pounds of it per year. Forty-eight pounds! Here are some of the proven benefits of kimchi:

- Gives rise to multiple probiotic strains of bacteria shown to survive stomach acid and provide health benefits in the colon.
- Lowers cholesterol.
- Promotes weight loss!
- Includes anti-inflammatory and potentially antiaging properties.
- Improves insulin sensitivity to prevent and reverse diabetes.
- Boosts multiple mechanisms by which it may protect us from cancer.

When it comes to eating kimchi, I love it for its spicy flavor but I'll readily admit it's not for everyone. My wife loves sauerkraut, but she'll never be a kimchi girl because she's not into spicy like I am. For me, I love kimchi as a condiment, or I like to throw it in a soup or rice bowl to add a unique flavor and extra spice. A little goes a long way.

Miso

I'm a *huge* miso fan! Miso is a paste made by fermenting soybeans with a fungus called *Aspergillus oryzae*. If you've never used it before, you have no clue what you're missing. It's both salty and savory at the same time, so it has a lot of umami. On a cold day it's so easy to just warm up some water and add a big scoop of miso to it for an impromptu miso soup. Even better if you have some fresh chives to cut on top and some seaweed to toss in. Miso offers:

- Protection from cancer. Miso may help prevent breast, colorectal, and liver cancer. This is actually a by-product of its soy content and the isoflavones, which are those scary "phytoestrogens" that some have vilified. It is important to set the record straight.
- And if you are worried about salt content and your blood pressure, fear not. Studies suggest miso *does not* raise blood pressure despite its salt content.
- Healthy bones! Calcium, vitamin K, and isoflavones all contribute to osteoporosis prevention.

Why drink an energy drink, another cup of coffee, or even tea when you could have a miso sipper for a healthy afternoon pick-me-up? You'll find this as one of the things we do during the Fiber Fueled 4 Weeks (see Chapter 10), but you can start today if you like. Simply purchase fermented organic miso. You'll find different colors—darker means stronger and saltier. White is sweeter, yellow has an earthy flavor, and red is bold with umami. I personally like red the most, but some recipes call for a gentler touch. Just add miso to warm water, stir until it dissolves into a beautiful broth, and drink! The key here is to add the miso when the water is lukewarm. If the water is scalding hot, then you'll kill the live bacteria in the miso. But if you add it to warm but not scalding water, you'll be good and still get the benefits.

Tempeh
Tempeh is another fermented soy product from Indonesia that has a nice, dense consistency and an earthy flavor. It's fun to cook with

tempeh because it tends to absorb the flavor of whatever spice or sauce that you throw at it. So what you have here is a versatile, delicious, and nutrient-dense food. The health benefits are the same as miso because tempeh is also made from fermented soybeans. It's really the way that tempeh can be used that makes it unique because it's a great source of protein that keeps its shape and can be steamed, pan-fried, blackened, or just crumbled raw over a salad or soup. It makes for great chili, stir-fries, sandwiches, stews, salads, and soups. One of my favorites is a tempeh Reuben, with nice dark rye bread, Thousand Island dressing, and some sauerkraut.

What about fermented dairy?

Why no love for kefir, yogurt, and other fermented dairy products? Let's look more closely at these foods. As we know, fermentation transforms our food and in many cases makes it easier to digest. This is particularly true with dairy products, where fermentation will remove most lactose. In fact, most hard cheeses, kefir, and yogurt are generally well tolerated by lactose-intolerant individuals. There are also some studies suggesting that kefir, yogurt, and other fermented dairy products may have health benefits. However, these studies were largely fraught with methodological limitations or were overtly paid for by the dairy industry.

So what are we supposed to make of corporate-sponsored research that is essentially a form of marketing and only being published because it makes the food look good and the conclusions are carefully guarded to protect the product? From my perspective, why take any risk when you can find delicious fermented nondairy yogurt and kefir? In particular, I love a coconut milk kefir that's available in Canada. No matter what you choose, make sure to pay attention to the sugar content, which is one of the big issues with all commercial products of this sort. Also, it should be noted that water kefir has absolutely nothing to do with milk and is much more similar to kombucha.

Sourdough bread

One of the things I love about sourdough bread is how simple it is to make. Just flour and water. Where's the yeast, you ask? It's true that baking bread generally requires baker's yeast, or *Saccharomyces cerevisiae*, for leavening. In the case of sourdough, you use a sourdough starter that contains a unique blend of wild yeast instead of the domesticated commercial yeast. Here's where it gets cool: You don't need to buy a starter if you don't want. Wild yeast is everywhere—in the air, in your flour, on the surface of grapes. So it's possible to use just water and flour to create your own starter, which will naturally be colonized by wild yeast to leaven your bread. But once you create a starter culture, you could use it pretty much forever. For example, the famous Boudin Bakery in San Francisco still uses the same yeast culture created by Isidore Boudin more than 170 years ago.

There are several other things I love about sourdough. First, it's delicious! I absolutely love that tangy flavor, soft bread, and flaky crust. Second, fermentation removes several of the antinutrients that some people worry about. For example, phytic acid is reduced by 62 percent. As we discussed earlier, sourdough also has less gluten and it's often better tolerated by those who are gluten intolerant. Finally, sourdough has a lower glycemic index compared to other types of bread, meaning that it causes less of a blood sugar spike and insulin response. I don't go out of my way to get more bread in my diet, but when I do eat bread I generally opt for sourdough. Rye and organic whole wheat can be great, too.

Kombucha

Kombucha is a fermented, lightly effervescent tea beverage that's all the rage. Sales are skyrocketing while people's health hopes are being hitched to this trendy beverage. I hate doing this, because I actually love kombucha, but we need to tone down our enthusiasm a little bit. Kombucha is not the lifesaving salve that people are hyping it up to be. And we shouldn't be guzzling it.

When you create kombucha, you start with old-fashioned sweet tea and introduce the right mix of bacteria and yeast. Those guys take over, consume the sugar, and transform the sweet tea into a tart, acidic beverage. In the process they construct a fibrous floating barrier at the surface called a SCOBY, standing for symbiotic culture of bacteria and yeast. It looks a little like a mushroom. I used to be scared of it. But then I started making my own kombucha, and have grown to adore and respect my SCOBY. People tend to hype up the "probiotics" in kombucha, but I actually love the other stuff—vitamins B_1, B_6, B_{12}, and C, antioxidant polyphenols, and healthy acids. Oh, and there's a little alcohol, but not enough that you'd drink kombucha for that reason although you should avoid it if you have a history of alcoholism.

While kombucha is a beverage that can be a part of a healthy diet, by itself it's not going to change your life. But nutrition is all about healthy substitutions. If you drop soda and replace it with a little kombucha, then you've done a good thing. And I absolutely love making my own kombucha at home and creating new flavors. I highly recommend it. You shouldn't drink more than 4 ounces in a day in my opinion, and I *always* dilute down my kombucha with water. It still has plenty of flavor but isn't quite so acidic. This helps alleviate one of the concerns of kombucha's acidity, which is that it can erode the enamel on your teeth.

■

I hope you see why fermented foods are an important part of the *Fiber Fueled* approach! Not only are they delicious but they're super-powered plant foods that have amazing healing abilities for your gut. If you don't eat many fermented foods now, have no fear. We're going to work them in nice and easy in my four-week plan. A little every day goes a long way. By the end you'll be in fermented nirvana, too.

To view the 45+ scientific references cited in this chapter, please visit me online at www.theplantfedgut.com/research/.

7

Prebiotics, Probiotics, and Postbiotics
Piecing together the "lesser biotics" to optimize your postbiotics (SCFAs)

I believe plants form the backbone of a healthy diet, and I whole-heartedly believe in the Golden Rule of maximizing plant-based diversity. Food comes first. Always.

But prebiotic and probiotic supplements can help accelerate the process of getting you *Fiber Fueled*, especially if digesting fiber is a challenge due to a damaged gut. The benefit of pre- and probiotic supplementation, particularly for anyone struggling with gut issues, is that we can augment the prebiotic fiber or healthy microbes in the gut in a targeted way without asking the gut to deal with anything else.

The healing effects can be profound and widespread. Pre- and pro-biotic supplements can improve our ability to process fiber and FODMAPs and also reduce the digestive distress that comes from dysbiosis and a damaged gut microbiome. Using our gut fitness anal-ogy, it's like working out your shoulders and feeling the effect of the shoulder workout when you bench-press. To properly train our gut, we need to start low and go slow with fiber and FODMAPs. Gut-health supplements can help. Let me show you.

The benefits of prebiotic supplements

Let's dive straight in. If you struggle with gut issues—bloating, flatulence, and so on—you might want to try a prebiotic supplement. Here are some of the positive outcomes we've seen in studies on prebiotic fiber supplementation:

- Growth of SCFA-producing gut microbes like *Bifidobacterium* and *Faecalibacterium prausnitzii*
- Reduced counts of unhealthy microbes such as *Bacteroides intestinalis*, *B. vulgatus*, and *Propionibacterium*
- Reduced bacterial endotoxin levels
- Reduced inflammatory markers like C-reactive protein, interleukin-6, or tumor necrosis factor
- Improvement in parameters of diabetes including lower postprandial blood sugar and insulin concentrations
- Lower total cholesterol
- Lower triglycerides
- Increased HDL cholesterol (the good cholesterol)
- Reduced fat mass
- Improved satiety with an increase in satiety hormones GLP-1 and peptide YY
- Improved absorption of calcium and magnesium

In a randomized, placebo-controlled trial of patients with IBS (both diarrhea and constipation variants included), researchers found that prebiotic galactooligosaccharides enhanced the growth of healthy gut bugs like *Bifidobacteria*, improved stool consistency to enhance bowel movement bliss, caused less flatulence and less bloating, and improved global symptoms of irritable bowel syndrome.

Now this is all well and good, but there's something interesting I found when I dug into the details of the study. They didn't just give people a single dose of a prebiotic and see what happened; they gave them one of two doses—low and high. What's interesting is that the lower dose of fiber actually produced more clinical improvement, meaning less bloating and less flatulence. How could this be? It comes back to our motto. When we're dealing with fiber and FODMAPs, low and slow is the way to grow. So when we introduce prebiotic supplements, more isn't necessarily better. Instead, let's start at a nice low dose and work our way up over time.

Choosing the right prebiotic for you

If you do decide to move forward with a prebiotic supplement, then the next question is "Which one?" We know from Chapter 3 that there are millions of types of fiber, and they're all different. Likewise, there are different formulations of prebiotic supplements and it is difficult to know which one exactly is going to be the right choice for you. It's about how that specific prebiotic interacts with the balance of gut microbes residing inside you.

With those thoughts in mind, here are a few favorites I use myself and with my patients:

- BETA GLUCANS: Found in oats, barley, wheat, and rye. Also found in seaweed and reishi, shiitake, and maitake mushrooms.
- PSYLLIUM: Comes from the outer coating, or "husk," of the plantago plant's seeds.
- PARTIALLY HYDROLYZED GUAR GUM: Derived from guar seed, a leguminous plant grown mainly in India and Pakistan.
- ACACIA POWDER: Made by grinding up acacia gum, a product of the acacia tree native to Africa. Can be taken in powder, capsule, or tablet form.
- WHEAT DEXTRIN: Most easily available. If you live in the United States you'll find this in virtually every drugstore or supermarket as Benefiber. Technically wheat dextrin is separated

from gluten, but since it is derived from wheat, I still have my patients with celiac or wheat allergy avoid this one.

- ISOMALTO-OLIGOSACCHARIDE (IMO): This is prebiotic fiber that's been prepared by fermentation. For example, you'll also find IMOs in miso, soy sauce, and honey. Makes it nice and gentle on the gut for the reasons we discussed in the previous chapter.

Each of these supplements is a natural prebiotic soluble fiber supplement derived from plants and offers some variety of health benefits commonly associated with prebiotics: promoting the growth of healthy gut microbes, release of postbiotic SCFAs, decrease in colon pH–inhibiting pathogenic bacteria, improvement of dysbiosis, correction of both diarrhea and constipation, lower cholesterol, blood sugar control, and protection against colorectal cancer. I've also found that these particular prebiotics are well tolerated relative to others. By comparison, there's a commonly used prebiotic called inulin out there. I've tried it a few times and every time I have noticed a substantial increase in gas and flatulence. So it's not my favorite.

Is one of these clearly superior to the others? No, I wouldn't say that. I've tried all of them and have also used them in countless patients, and my experience has shown me that the fiber interacts with your unique, personal gut microbiota and so different people respond differently. The key is to experiment.

The way you add these into your diet is not complicated—it doesn't matter that much what time you take them unless you have diabetes or high cholesterol. In that case, you'll want to take them with meals. The more important thing is to take them consistently and to start slow and low and work your way up to tolerance. Start with one dosage a day to ease your body into it. I like to get my daily dose of prebiotics in my morning coffee. They are soluble fiber and so they dissolve in liquid easily. You honestly don't even know they're there.

The last thing is to remember that the one Golden Rule—plant-based diversity—applies to your prebiotics, too. I personally like to mix several different types of prebiotics into my week, so I can get the gut-building benefits of each. But in the very beginning, particularly if you have a damaged gut, you want to start low, go slow, and only do one fiber supplement at a time so you train up your gut with one type of fiber at a time.

Probiotics: Hype with a sprinkle of science

Let's look at our formula again for a moment:

$$\textbf{prebiotics + probiotics = postbiotics}$$

Okay, we've got prebiotics covered in our diet and supplements—check. We also get an increase in probiotic bacteria by fiber fueling our colon with plant-based diversity. Double check. But the million-dollar question is: Can we amp this healing up to an even higher level with a probiotic supplement?

So what exactly are probiotics? Well, they are live microorganisms—generally bacteria and/or yeast. But they're not just any old live micro-organisms. By definition, probiotics are live microorganisms that, when administered in adequate amounts, you guessed it: "confer a health benefit on the host." The theory with probiotics is that they mimic the effects of our intact microbiota. In other words, just like our healthy gut microbes, these probiotics should optimize our im-mune system, reduce inflammation, inhibit the growth of pathogenic bacteria, correct leaky gut and restore gut barrier integrity, reestablish intestinal motility, and even improve mood. We've seen probiotics work this way in animal models, but do they translate to humans?

Right off the bat, let me say that the hype around probiotics is out-pacing the science big time. Sadly, probiotics have gotten popular because of marketing and because they are what everyone wants—a new pill that's cutting edge, ideally natural, that will require zero effort and fix all your problems. But the truth is that you can't fix a bad diet with a probiotic. You can't go low carb, low fiber, and fix your gut with a probiotic. Returning to our formula: You can't get to postbiotics without prebiotics. And you can't optimize plant-based diversity by getting all of your fiber from a supplement. It just doesn't work that way. It's time to move past "biohacking" and realize that there are no shortcuts.

It's also important to know that probiotics don't stick. In other words, they generally don't colonize your gut permanently, mostly because you already have a community of bacteria in place and they're resistant to newcomers. You're not adding back new bacteria or ones you lost. If you stop taking the probiotic, then within two to five days it'll be like you never took it in the first place. So the effects of probiotics appear to occur as they transiently pass through the intestine. But along the way, they're working their magic, including helping to unleash SCFAs from our prebiotics. They do give our innate microbes a helping hand, but then they disappear.

Fermented foods vs. probiotics

What's the difference between fermented foods and probiotics? They both contain live bacteria, but beyond that they are very different. A probiotic is a highly concentrated version of a limited number of bacterial strains, usually delivered by a capsule of some sort. Fermented foods, on the other hand, are living foods that have a wider variety of microorganisms but in lower numbers. But with the fermented food you also get all the other good stuff—exopolysaccharide prebiotics, vitamins, healthy acids, bioactive peptides, and polyphenols—all of which are also providing benefit. Sometimes you need the concentrated focus of

PREBIOTICS, PROBIOTICS, AND POSTBIOTICS 143

specific bacterial strains to give your gut a boost, and that's when
you need a probiotic. Eating fermented foods regularly should be
a part of your long-term plan to promote a healthy gut.

The science to support probiotics

It may sound like I don't believe in probiotics at all, but I recommend
them in my clinic every day, often with great results. Without a doubt,
some of you reading this book would benefit from them. Let's jump
into the science first; then I'll explain how to use probiotics effectively.

Probiotics often help with digestive symptoms and have been
shown to improve abdominal pain, bloating, diarrhea, constipation,
and other symptoms of irritable bowel syndrome. In inflammatory
bowel disease, probiotics have shown benefit for patients with ulcerative colitis and pouchitis. So far there aren't any good studies of benefit in Crohn's disease.

Should you take probiotics after antibiotics? The answer may surprise you.

Probiotics are known to treat antibiotic-associated diarrhea in
adults. They also protect against developing *Clostridioides difficile*
infection. For years I was a believer that the best way to recover
from antibiotic use was to take a probiotic for a few weeks. But a
recent study has completely changed my mind. In it, researchers
from Israel showed convincingly that probiotics actually impair
the microbiota's ability to stabilize and return to normal after
antibiotics. They actually slow recovery. So unless directly
recommended by a doctor, I avoid probiotics immediately after
antibiotics. Instead, focus on your diet first. Maximize plant-based

diversity. Then add in prebiotics to help your gut microbes bounce back faster. Avoid chemicals, saturated fat, and pesticides in your food. No alcohol. Exercise and get into nature. Go to bed early and sleep at least eight hours. And most important, let's avoid unnecessary antibiotic use.

We previously learned that prebiotic galacto-oligosaccharides can improve lactose digestion, providing evidence that strengthening the gut can also improve our capacity to process and digest our food. Using our gut fitness analogy, that's like working out your shoulders and then discovering that your bench press got stronger. In similar fashion, we find that probiotics can also improve our ability to process lactose. This is important because it suggests that the digestive enzymes in probiotics may be able to help us break down our carbohydrates and get the benefits.

There are now numerous studies to suggest that probiotics may be beneficial for intestinal bloating. Some specific strains that have been shown to be beneficial in studies include *Lactobacillus plantarum*, *Bifidobacterium infantis*, *L. acidophilus*, and *Bifidobacterium lactis*. Even a group of healthy people reported that their bowel movements were more blissful when they were using a daily probiotic.

A more targeted role for probiotics

So yes, probiotics actually do something. Are they a silver bullet as they're marketed at times to be, capable of fixing all of our problems? Nope. That is hype rather than science. Separating fact from fiction requires us to get smart and understand how probiotics work, and also learn how to be smart shoppers so we can pick the best one for us.

Let's start here . . . diet always comes first. The average human eats eighty thousand pounds of food during their lifetime, and a supplement will never overcome a bad diet. But in pre- and probiotics are an additional tool to help you optimize SCFA levels and restore gut health. Here's what to prioritize:

1. The Golden Rule—Diversity of Plants
2. Prebiotics
3. Probiotics

I can't wait for the day when we can analyze a person's individual microbiome, identify the strengths and weaknesses, and then give them the exact strains in the exact proportions that they need for optimal health or to fix a problem. Studies are starting to emerge showing us that probiotic colonization can be personalized. But unfortunately, that day has not arrived yet. So the current reality is that we're shooting in the dark. We're choosing a probiotic blindly without knowing how it fits with our completely personal, unique microbiota. We can only hope that it'll match, but it doesn't always work that way. So we *have* to accept a trial-and-error element. If it works and you notice a difference, stick with it. If it doesn't, move on. It may be the best probiotic in the world, but it doesn't mean it's the best probiotic for you.

Should everyone be taking a pre- and probiotic?

Are there benefits to prebiotics and probiotics in a healthy population, meaning: Do they boost your health if you are not taking them to address any specific symptom or health issue? I would argue that prebiotics provide more benefit in this circumstance. In normal, healthy adults, prebiotics have still been shown to improve metabolic parameters. For example, they help regulate blood sugar after meals, lower insulin concentrations (improved insulin sensitivity), and increase satiety to make you feel full faster. I use a prebiotic most days. I'm committed to the Golden Rule, so I often rotate through several types. There are definitely days that I forget it, and I notice a difference. When I'm taking it, my bowel movements are glorious. I'll just leave it at that.

As for probiotics, a comprehensive review found that they reduced the incidence, duration, and symptoms of the common cold (but not influenza), suggesting an immune benefit. There was minimal effect on metabolic parameters such as cholesterol level, weight, blood sugar, or insulin with probiotics.

When considering whether or not prebiotics and probiotics make sense in the absence of disease, there are two additional considerations. One is safety. Both have been used widespread for decades now by the general population and the safety record has been excellent in both health and disease. There are case reports of infectious complications with probiotics, one study with increased risk if probiotics are given to someone with severe acute pancreatitis and one series where probiotics caused reversible brain fog in a population with severe motility disorders. This may sound scary, but consider the millions of people taking a probiotic on a daily basis for decades now and that these possibilities are at the most extremely rare. It goes without saying that you should discuss these issues with your doctor and obviously stop any medicine or supplement that you believe is causing an adverse effect. But that said, the safety record of both pre- and probiotics is very good.

The second consideration is cost. Prebiotics are not very expensive, but a good probiotic is around $40. Sure, you can find $5 probiotics at the store, but they're so impotent you'd be better off buying a tub of sauerkraut. So it's up to you and what works best with your budget. Until proven otherwise, I'm a bigger believer in prebiotic supplementation over probiotics if you're healthy and trying to stay that way.

If you are trying to figure out where to start with a probiotic, start with this question: What are you trying to accomplish? Do you have a specific symptom that you're trying to alleviate? You should have a reason that you're opting to take a probiotic, and if you don't or it's simply, "I want a healthier gut," then food is best. Remember, every plant has its own microbiome. So when we eat them, there's a sharing of microbes that occurs, and that's one advantage of consuming living food. When we opt for a little fermented food every day, we're taking that to the next level.

But if you have an answer to the question, "What are you trying to accomplish?" you'll want to find some studies that have been done to see if there's something out there that's known to work best for your specific issue. You can head to my website, www.theplantfedgut.com, where I've got lots of resources and support for how to research and choose a probiotic that's best for you. Here's the key: You want to find the probiotic that fits your treatment goal. You can do this by finding a study that shows a benefit, and then choosing that probiotic and using it the way they did in the study. For example, if you're trying to correct constipation, then you'd look for a probiotic with *Bifidobacterium lactis* in at least 17.2 billion colony-forming units (the unit of measurement for number of bacteria) because that's what worked for constipation in a placebo-controlled trial.

Beyond looking at studies for guidance on which probiotic and at what dose, I'm a big believer in quality. Here's a list of the things I look for in assessing whether a probiotic is of sufficient quality:

Quantity of bacteria: More is generally better. Typically I look for 25 billion to 50 billion minimum if trying to correct a medical issue.

Number of individual strains: Again, more is better. We know that bacteria work in "guilds" or teams, so it's better to have a diverse team than to pretend these bacteria work in isolation.

Now, which bacteria you need for a specific disease are to be determined, but until then we know that multistrain probiotics tend to outperform single-strain probiotics.

Guaranteed quantity at expiration: The packaging should define not just how many bacteria there are at the time of manufacture, but how many are guaranteed by a defined expiration date. This is a marker of probiotic quality and, if absent, raises concerns.

Allergen free: I prefer my probiotic to be free of dairy, eggs, nuts, seafood, soy, wheat, and gluten. While we're on the topic, I personally want my probiotic to be vegan. This ensures that it's not dairy based, which many of the probiotics on the market are.

Delayed-release capsule: We need to get the probiotics to the area in your body where the bacteria actually live, which is in the colon. Without a special delayed-release capsule, many of them will be destroyed by your stomach acid.

Packaging and need for refrigeration: Let me say this: I generally refrigerate anyway. But it's a sign of improved survivability of the probiotic if it does not *require* refrigeration. I love my probiotics in blister packs, which means that each individual capsule is protected from bacteria-damaging humidity.

When will the future of probiotics arrive?

Knowing which bacterial strains to combine in our probiotics is the challenge. Again, we know that microbes function as teams, or "guilds." We need to figure out how to build the proper team to accomplish our specific goal. It's an incredibly challenging process to engineer because we're talking about measuring hundreds of species, which dynamically change by the millisecond, differ by anatomical geography, and interact with each other and their environment. But the probiotic engineered by nature over three million years already contains those guilds and that balance. Yes, I'm talking about POOP! We disrespect and overlook it, but it may be the savior of modern medicine. There are dozens of active clinical trials evaluating the role of fecal transplant in human health. My prediction is that fecal transplant will be more effective for acute illnesses (like infection) than for chronic illnesses (like colitis or Crohn's disease) and that concurrent lifestyle changes are needed to support the newly received microbiota. I'm excited to see what the studies find!

To view the 35+ scientific references cited in this chapter, please visit me online at www.theplantfedgut.com/research/.

8

The Fiber Fueled Foods

*Inspiring your gut microbes to do
the* Riverdance *at every meal*

You may have noticed that our food culture is obsessed with "super-foods." We're all looking for that one game changer that's going to fix all of our health problems and make us feel like a million bucks. We're encouraged to reach for pills we can pop to make everything better. Minimal effort with maximum results. Don't get me wrong, superfoods (and medications, when you need them) are great. But we got it a little twisted because no *one* food is capable of meeting that expectation. There aren't three hundred thousand plants on Earth so that we could pick just one and gorge ourselves on it.

There's no perfect food—they all have strengths and weaknesses. I'm the first to admit that there are weaknesses to the healthy foods I'm promoting in this book. It goes back to our conversation from Chapter 4. Too much of a good thing can hurt you. If all you ate was kale, you would be *incredibly* unhealthy.

When we focus on superfoods alone, we miss out on diversity of plants. Superfoods are cool, but I will take plant-based diversity over superfoods every day of the week.

Remember that food is not just a bunch of individual components, it's an entire package. Do the benefits outweigh the negatives? Bring food into your life that's more positive than negative. When we do that, we get the best from our diet. That's where plant-based diversity comes in—each plant might not be individually perfect, but the positives far outweigh the negatives, and when you consider them collectively you have a diet perfectly tailored to support a healthy gut microbiota and overall health.

That said, we can focus on diversity of plants and at the same time incorporate foods that are true nutritional powerhouses to get the best of both those worlds. These turbocharged foods can be our "best friends," but they shouldn't be our only friends.

Here are my favorite Fiber Fueled foods, conveniently organized into an acronym to make them easy to remember. These are the foods I try to sneak in as often as possible, but they are most powerful in combination and when you eat them with more plant varieties.

F GOALS

F: Fruit & Fermented
G: Greens & Grains
O: Omega-3 Super Seeds
A: Aromatics (onions, garlic)
L: Legumes
S: Sulforaphane (broccoli sprouts and other cruciferous veggies)

F: Fruit & Fermented

In Chapter 6, we celebrated fermented foods for their increased nutritional value, prebiotics, probiotics, and enrichment with postbiotics. They also add further plant-based diversity to our diet. Remember that our goal is to add a small serving of fermented foods to our daily routine.

But there's a second "F" in our F GOALS and that's fruit. There's an inordinate amount of fear of fruit out there, particularly in the fitness community where I've seen or heard many personal trainers say, "Fruit has sugar, and excess sugar can lead to weight gain." Folks, we shouldn't look at any food only through the lens of its individual components because it will cause us to make conclusions that are flat-out wrong. We need to look at whole foods. The sugar in fruit is by no means the same as processed sugar. It's packed in with everything else in the fruit, including vitamins and minerals, phytochemicals, and *fiber*.

And no, eating whole fruit does not cause "weight gain." It's actually quite the opposite. It doesn't cause diabetes, either, for that matter. Instead, it actually can protect against it. For example, as sweet as berries may be, they actually lower blood sugar and insulin release after a meal. Whether you are diabetic or looking to avoid sugar for another reason, don't make the mistake of lumping natural sugar in whole fruit in with added or processed sugars. You absolutely should be eating fruit! It can help you lose weight and control your diabetes.

What about juicing?

Is juiced fruit the same as sinking your teeth into the whole food? No, unfortunately, it's not. When you process your food, the rules no longer apply. When you juice your fruit, you are removing most of the fiber and artificially concentrating the sugar. For example, one small orange has 45 calories, 2.3 grams of fiber, and 9 grams of sugars. One cup of OJ packs in 134 calories, just 0.5 gram of fiber, and 23.3 grams of sugars. Fruit juice is a sugar beverage, created by the manipulation of a whole food.

I could write an entire book about the health benefits you'll find in fruit. In Chapter 4 we learned that apples are an excellent source of prebiotic fiber, healthy microbes, and numerous beneficial polyphenol phytochemicals contributing to reduced risk of heart disease, stroke, lung cancer, diabetes, asthma, and weight loss. Oranges have vitamin C and antioxidant flavonoids and anthocyanins that protect against hypertension, high cholesterol, kidney stones, and iron deficiency. Nice, right?

So apples and oranges are great, but let me tell you about my deep and abiding love for *berries*: blueberries, blackberries, raspberries, strawberries, and the lesser known acai and goji berries. Give me all of them!

Berries come in incredible colors: blue, purple, red, and pink. The color actually comes from a phytochemical (remember, "phyto" means "plant-based") called anthocyanins. Without anthocyanins, blueberries would be green! That's why immature blueberries aren't blue, because the anthocyanins haven't come in yet. Anthocyanins are pretty magical. They help protect against cancer, and they also boost cognition. For example, in one study women who ate just two servings of strawberries or one serving of blueberries per week postponed cognitive decline and made their brain behave like it was thirty months younger. In another study, two servings of berries a week yielded a 23 percent less chance of developing Parkinson's. And when wild blueberries were given to kids, they saw almost immediate improvements in cognitive performance that increased based upon the dose of blueberries. I recently took a grueling eight-hour exam to renew my board certification in internal medicine. Guess what I was eating all day? Blueberries.

Pro Tip: Blueberries
Opt for the smaller blueberries, ideally wild. Smaller blueberries are less sweet but have higher levels of antioxidants.

But let's not ignore the fiber content. In a one-cup serving of straw-berries, blueberries, blackberries, and raspberries, you'll find 3, 4, 8, and 8 grams of fiber in each, respectively. Considering that the average American is only getting 15 or 16 grams of fiber in a day, a simple handful of berries can make a big difference. I love popping a couple of handfuls of berries as an afternoon snack or when I have a sweet tooth.

G: Greens & Grains

In Chapter 4 we discussed the merits of whole grains, such as reduced risk of coronary heart disease, cardiovascular disease, and total cancer as well as lower likelihood of death from all causes, respiratory dis-eases, infectious diseases, diabetes, and all non-cardiovascular, non-cancer causes. That was just one study.

It's pretty straightforward from my perspective. Drop the refined grains, no doubt. I'm with you 100 percent. But if you want a healthy microbiota, whole grains are at the foundation of building a healthy gut. And the numerous studies cited in Chapter 4 support it.

There's a second important "G" in the house, and that's greens. There is so much plant-based diversity when it comes to greens: col-lards, kale, arugula, spinach, romaine, bok choy, watercress, Swiss chard, broccoli raab, mustard greens, sorrel, escarole, kohlrabi, and more. And there are varieties within these foods, too. For example, kale varieties include curly, lacinato (aka dinosaur or Tuscan kale), Redbor, or Siberian. Even the leaves of some favorite root veggies like beet, turnip, dandelion, radish, and carrots are edible and offer more variety in the green category.

When we assess the health benefits of food, nutrient density is a key concept. The idea is to get the maximum amount of nutrients—vitamins, minerals, phytochemicals, fiber—per calorie consumed. This becomes a simple formula: nutrient density equals nutrients di-vided by calories. So if you think about oil, for example, it's high in calories and low in nutrients. Poor nutrient density. Or potato chips. High in calories, low in nutrients. This is a pretty straightforward, logical approach, right?

We call it the ANDI score, which stands for Aggregate Nutrient Density Index and was developed by the legendary Dr. Joel Fuhrman, one of my personal health heroes. The score is from 1 to 1,000, with 1 being the worst. For example, cola, corn chips, and vanilla ice cream got the lowest score. Sounds about right. As for the high performers, there were five with a perfect 1,000 score—kale, collards, mustard greens, watercress, and Swiss chard. Bok choy, spinach, arugula, and romaine were the next four highest scores. In other words, greens were the top nine foods on the list. This wasn't a list restricted to just greens. All foods were eligible, yet greens hold a monopoly at the top.

The absurd amount of nutrient density in greens is a present from Mother Nature. You get tons of nutrients packaged with almost no calories, so you can literally eat as much as you want. It's getting your nutrients served without the calories! For example, an entire pound of leafy greens has only 100 calories. That's about one egg or two bites of steak. I've stopped worrying about portion size ever since I transitioned to a plant-based diet, but if you do continue to consume high-calorie foods after reading this book, know that you can throw unlimited amounts of greens in there to get more nutrients in your diet without compromising calories.

Let's highlight a few examples of this nutrient density hard at work:

- **Kale:** Kale contains antioxidant phytochemicals lutein and zeaxanthin, which are required by the eyes to prevent macular degeneration. It also contains beta-carotene, which reduces the risk of getting cataracts.
- **Collard greens:** You can't live in Charleston, South Carolina, and not love collard greens. But what's beautiful is that they can sneak nutrients in on even the most unsuspecting Southern

palate. Turns out that collards bind bile acids in the intestines and eliminate them in our stool. This helps to lower cholesterol and reduces carcinogenic secondary bile acids.

Pro Tip: Greens
Steam your greens to improve bile salt–binding activity! This helps protect against cancer, specifically colon and liver cancer.

- **Spinach:** You may recall that Popeye got his superhuman strength by popping a can of spinach. Popeye was created in 1929, so this was incredibly forward-thinking. And it's true! Just one cup of cooked spinach offers 36 percent of your daily value for iron and 11 percent for protein, not to mention a bonus of vitamins A and K, calcium, magnesium, potassium, and manganese. Oh, and 4 grams of fiber.
- **Arugula:** Arugula is a cancer destroyer. It has a unique mix of phytochemicals like thiocyanates, sulforaphane, and indoles that may help fight some of our most deadly cancers—prostate, breast, colon, ovarian, and cervical. We'll come back to sulforaphane in a minute.
- **Bok choy:** Bok choy is great for your bones, offering critical minerals like iron, zinc, and magnesium in combination with vitamin K.
- **Romaine:** If you're looking for healthy skin and to reverse aging, grab some romaine. The vitamins A and C in romaine help to lay down fresh collagen to prevent wrinkles and neutralize oxidizing free radicals. The result is glowing, radiant skin with improved elasticity.

O: Omega-3 Super Seeds

I absolutely adore this category because I feel like these foods have it all—they are nutritious, delicious, versatile, and unique. But before I jump in, a few words on omega-3 and omega-6 fatty acids. You've heard of different fat types: trans, saturated, monounsaturated, polyunsaturated. These omega-3 and -6 fats are polyunsaturated fats, and they're considered "essential" because our body is not capable of intrinsically making them so we are required to get them from our diet. If you don't consume them, you develop a deficiency, which can lead to sickness.

Generally speaking, polyunsaturated fats are considered healthy and are important for many functions in the body. But you've probably heard about omega-3s more than omega-6s. Part of the reason why you've heard so much about omega-3s is that the modern Western diet provides an excessive amount of omega-6s and an inadequate amount of omega-3s. The ratio of omega-6s to omega-3s is a marker of health. Traditional cultures are thought to have evolved with a nearly even mix between omega-6s and omega-3s, while most Westerners are functioning with a ratio between 15 and 16.7 to 1 of excess omega-6s. It's a ratio that when skewed can promote disease: cardiovascular disease, cancer, osteoporosis, and autoimmune diseases. Our goal is to balance this ratio, which means that we need an influx of omega-3s in our diet.

And I know just where we can find them—omega-3 super seeds. To be specific, I'm referring to three types of seeds that contain plant-based omega-3s: flaxseeds, chia seeds, and hemp seeds. While each offers the omega-3s, there are differences between each so let's break it down a little bit.

- **Flaxseed:** Flaxseeds are an excellent source of omega-3 alpha-linolenic acid (ALA), with 2,300 milligrams of ALA per tablespoon of flax. But it is also an excellent source of soluble fiber, which is part of the reason why it's a traditional remedy for constipation. You get all the goodness that comes with prebiotic fiber as discussed in Chapter 3. Flax is also particularly rich in lignans, which are plant chemicals that strongly protect against hormonal cancers like breast and prostate cancer.

Pro Tip: Flaxseed

Flaxseeds have a hard shell and must be ground or thoroughly chewed in order for their nutrients to be absorbed. If you buy pre-ground flax, simply keep it in your freezer to maintain freshness.

- **Chia seeds:** You'll find lignans in chia seeds as well, though the levels are higher in flax. Chia has ever so slightly more omega-3s (2,400 vs. 2,300 milligrams per tablespoon) and significantly more fiber (5 grams in chia vs. 3 grams in flax). Chia seeds are 40 percent fiber by weight, making them one of the top sources of fiber in the world. This is mostly soluble fiber, which is the prebiotic kind. You can see the soluble fiber on display if you stir a tablespoon of chia into a quarter cup of liquid and within ten minutes you'll find a viscous gel. Chia seeds can absorb ten to twelve times their weight in water. Let them sit in water for a few hours and you'll make chia pudding, which is nutritious and has a texture resembling tapioca pudding.

- **Hemp seeds:** Last but not least are hemp seeds. They're, ahem, different from flax and chia. Okay, let me just get this out of the way. Yes, hemp seeds come from the same plant as marijuana. But they're legal! They don't contain THC, the psychoactive part of cannabis. So they won't get you high, but they *will* get you healthy. Hemps seeds have about 40 percent of the omega-3 ALA that you find in chia and flax, but less fiber. When you think of hemp seeds, think of protein. Hemp seeds are unique in that they are complete protein, meaning they contain all of the essential amino

acids. So hemp seeds are a one-stop shop for both essential fats
and amino acids.

■

I love throwing omega-3 super seeds in my smoothie. Honestly, I'll
often put all three in at the same time. They go well with oatmeal or
in some cases on a fresh salad. And you'll find a mouthwatering recipe
for chia pudding (Zesty Lemon Chia Pudding, page 251) in Chapter
10, "The Fiber Fueled 4 Weeks."

There are a few other sources of plant-based omega-3s to be aware
of—walnuts, firm tofu, and edamame have a decent amount of ALA,
although much less than flax or chia. Beans and Brussels sprouts have
a small amount, as well.

A: Aromatics (Onions, Garlic)

These are the flavor foods! Think of a heavenly, slow-simmered Italian sauce heavily laden with garlic, onions, and basil.

Always add fresh herbs

Herbs are incredibly nutrient-dense. Basil alone has numerous
phytochemicals, giving it anti-inflammatory, chemo-preventive, radio-
protective, antimicrobial, analgesic, antipyretic, antidiabetic,
hepatoprotective, hypolipidemic, and immunomodulatory properties. Here's
my point: Any time you have the opportunity to add fresh herbs and spices to
a dish, do it! You're adding flavor, plant-based diversity, and multiple
phytochemicals.

The great flavor that you get with onions and garlic is because
they're both allium vegetables. Others in this category with similar
benefits are leeks, shallots, chives, and scallions. At baseline, allium
vegetables are jam-packed with nutrients: vitamins B_1, B_2, B_3, B_6, C, E,
K, folate, iron, magnesium, phosphorus, sodium, and zinc. Jam. Packed.

But then we get into the really good stuff. Allium contains aromatic organosulfur compounds that are responsible for their smell, their taste, and their health benefits. For example, when fresh garlic or onions are chopped or crushed, an enzyme called alliinase is activated and converts alliin into allicin. It takes ten minutes for the enzyme to activate the allicin, a compound that has antibacterial, antifungal, antiparasitic, and even antiviral properties. The stronger the smell, the better it is for your health. To allow allicin to activate, *CHOP, then STOP* and wait for ten minutes before cooking with alliums. The allicin appears to target the bad guys like multidrug-resistant enterotoxigenic *E. coli* and *Candida albicans.* And it promotes the growth of *Bifidobacteria* and other healthy microbes in the gut. It's worth noting that alliums are also an excellent source of prebiotic fiber.

Garlic: my secret weapon in the fight against the common cold
In our family we have a tradition of using garlic to fight the common cold. At the first sign of a sore throat, we start ingesting garlic. Basically, we will cut two to four garlic cloves into pill-size pieces. CHOP then STOP. Wait ten minutes for the alliinase to activate the allicin, then swallow whole. I'll do this daily until the cold is gone, and I've actually reversed colds by consuming the garlic pieces when I just start to feel symptoms. There's a placebo controlled trial that supports my experience. But you do smell a little like garlic while you're talking. Small price to pay.

Allium veggies also have potent anticancer activity, particularly against gastric and prostate cancer. There are two layers to the anticancer activity. First, the organosulfur compounds like allicin detoxify carcinogens, block tumor growth, and prevent blood flow to the tumor. Second, allium veggies contain at least twenty-four different flavonoid phytochemicals, such as quercetin. Red onions have the added benefit of anthocyanidins. The flavonoids have anti-inflammatory effects that may help protect us from cancer.

These antioxidant compounds also appear to be beneficial for Alzheimer's dementia and heart disease.

Pro Tip: Onions

When you chop an onion, you set off a reaction creating the organosulfides that makes your eyes tear. These are the cancer-fighting and anti-inflammatory compounds, so we embrace them. If you tear up when cutting your onion, try throwing the onion in the freezer for five minutes to make it cold before cutting. To get the most out of your allium veggies, it's ideal to eat them raw but if not, cut them and let them sit to form the compounds before cooking. (CHOP, then STOP.)

L: Legumes

Legumes are among the healthiest foods on the planet. And they are dirt cheap! They are at the foundation of a healthy gut microbiota, offering prebiotic fiber and resistant starches in spades. Please don't pass up the opportunity to build your gut on these irreplaceable foods. See Chapter 4 for more information on legumes.

S: Sulforaphane (Broccoli Sprouts and Other Cruciferous Veggies)

Plants are like my children. I love all of them, and I can see the beauty in their individuality. But if there's one I love the most, this is the one. I have been waiting eight chapters to talk to you about cruciferous vegetables and their super chemical *sulforaphane*.

We all know broccoli, kale, arugula, cabbage, cauliflower, and Brussels sprouts as healthy foods. But what's so special about them? They're part of a family of vegetables that we refer to as cruciferous. There are at least forty family members, but they share a common lineage. Through billions of years of plant evolution, they evolved a common defense system using an enzyme called myrosinase to convert glucosinolates into "toxic" compounds. The myrosinase and glucosinolates are stored in separate compartments within the plant, so under normal circumstances they don't mix. But when an insect or invading herbivore—like yours truly—starts mashing on the plant, they'll break the separating chambers, mix the chemicals, and set off a chemical reaction leading to the production of isothiocyanates (ITCs) like sulforaphane. It's conceptually similar to a bomb. So what happens when the bomb goes off and these ITCs are released? Cancer is cured, inflammation is squashed, hearts get healthy, blood sugar comes down, fat gets burned, and hormones get balanced. ITCs are powerfully health promoting. This is yet another example where a plant's defense mechanism can also do double duty as *our* defense against cancer cells.

Pro Tip: Cruciferous Vegetables

Cruciferous veggies are similar to onions and garlic in that they have an enzyme that needs to be activated to get the most healing benefits and therefore are best consumed raw. Similar to the aromatics, you can employ the CHOP then STOP technique to activate the enzyme prior to cooking or eating. If the broccoli or cauliflower has already been cooked, as happens with frozen vegetables that have been heat blanched prior to freezing, you can replace some of the enzyme that has been lost and restore the healing isothiocyanate phytochemicals by sprinkling mustard seed powder on the vegetables after cooking. A cool trick!

Let's talk about my favorite isothiocyanate—sulforaphane. You get sulforaphane from cruciferous vegetables like broccoli, Brussels sprouts, kale, and cabbage. In 1992, Dr. Paul Talalay, a true pioneer in the field of cancer prevention, opened Pandora's box when he first published on the cancer protective effects of sulforaphane. Since that time there have been hundreds of laboratory, animal, and some human studies (many by Dr. Talalay himself, who recently passed away at age ninety-five) suggesting that sulforaphane may be the driving force behind these incredibly healthy foods. Here's what we have learned about sulforaphane, this medicinal phytochemical:

- Protects us from cancer by seven mechanisms: inhibits the production of carcinogens, activates enzymes to detoxify the carcinogens that are produced, shuts down blood flow to the tumor (which is needed to fuel growth), inhibits cancer cell migration and invasion, promotes self-destruction of cancer cells (apoptosis), and even regulates cancer development through epigenetics.
- Undermines lung, colon, breast, prostate, skin, pancreatic, liver, throat, and bladder cancer, osteosarcoma, glioblastoma, leukemia, melanoma—and potentially more.
- Shuts down the pro-inflammatory pathways that get activated by bacterial endotoxin.
- Works as a powerful antioxidant to detoxify free radicals and reduce cellular damage.
- May benefit Parkinson's, and recovery from stroke, concussion, or other brain trauma.
- Reduces amyloid beta plaques and improves cognitive impairment in Alzheimer's patients.
- Improves mood, as well as anxiety and depression.
- Boosts brain function, improving memory and focus.
- Regulates the immune system, ameliorating autoimmune diseases like experimental multiple sclerosis and rheumatoid arthritis.
- Flips the body into fat-burning mode to promote weight loss, amazingly by reducing pathogenic bad bacteria in the gut and limiting bacterial endotoxin release in addition to other mechanisms.
- Combats bacterial and fungal infections. In one study, twenty-three out of twenty-eight pathogenic bacterial and fungal species were inhibited.

- Protects the heart by improving lipids, lowering blood pressure, inhibiting platelet aggregation, and even directly suppressing inflammation in the arteries.
- Improves insulin sensitivity to correct type 2 diabetes.
- Repairs the damage of diabetes, correcting diabetic heart and kidney damage.
- Protects the liver and kidneys from the damage done by some chemotherapeutic drugs.

Believe it or not, I could keep going. So how does sulforaphane interact with our gut microbiota? We saw above that sulforaphane is capable of reducing levels of pathogenic bacteria and bacterial endotoxin release. But there's so much more. In another study, sulforaphane corrected gut dysbiosis by increasing healthy gut microbes, *increasing butyrate release*, and repairing the intestinal lining to reverse leaky gut by upregulating tight junction formation. Mind. Blown. What I'm saying here is that part of the way sulforaphane works its absolute magic is by tag teaming with SCFAs to create the most powerful gut-healing superhero duo of all time.

It's all about the cruciferous veggies, specifically broccoli, Brussels sprouts, cabbage, cauliflower, and kale. But there is one food that *dominates* all others in terms of offering more sulforaphane: *broccoli sprouts*. These are essentially immature broccoli, where the seed has just recently hatched and we have the earliest thing beyond a seed. The concept is the same as bean sprouts or alfalfa sprouts. Broccoli sprouts can produce ten to one hundred times more sulforaphane than mature broccoli. What this means is that you can either eat massive quantities of fully mature broccoli or a small amount of broccoli sprouts and achieve the same effect.

Grow your own broccoli sprouts! It's easy.

- Add 2 tablespoons of broccoli sprouting seeds to a wide-mouthed 1-quart mason jar.
- Cover with 2 inches of filtered water and cap with a sprouting lid. Store in a warm, dark place, like the kitchen cabinet, overnight. In the morning you're going to drain the water. This is the only time you're going to leave the seeds submerged in water. From here on out it'll be rinse and drain.
- Rinse the seeds with fresh water two or three times per day. Swirl, then drain the water. It's important to get most of the water out, so one strategy is to place the mason jar upside down in a large bowl so that it's at a 45-degree angle (or so) so the drops can continue to fall out. Again, this is the process you're repeating two or three times daily—rinse, swirl, drain, rest in the cabinet, repeat.

    Over the course of days you will see changes: first they break open and grow (so cute!), then they extend to be an inch or so long with yellow leaves. At this point, it's time for them to get some sunlight. Sunlight will help them mature, the leaves will turn green, and you are done! Cover them with an airtight seal and store in the fridge.

Broccoli sprouts have a bitter, peppery flavor, but it's that bitterness that is blasting cancer cells on your behalf. And note: Taking a supplement instead just can't match the effect of the broccoli sprouts. In a study comparing broccoli sprouts to a supplement, the real thing dominated. Whole foods win, yet again! If the taste bothers you, try using broccoli sprouts in a smoothie, soup, or larger salad.

Bonus: Shrooms & Seaweed

I'm pretty sure you now understand why sulforaphane deserved its own category. Honestly, there may be no single food that represents the idea of "Food Is Medicine" better than broccoli sprouts. But mushrooms and seaweed deserve a quick shout-out as a bonus category.

Shrooms deserve mention because they are entirely unique—they're not even plants! They're fungi, but let's make them honorary plants because they sure behave as such. They contain prebiotic beta-glucan, which strengthens the immune system to prevent infections and even cancer. Several types even offer unique protection against breast cancer. Eating one button mushroom per day is associated with a 64 percent reduction in breast cancer risk. One beautiful thing about mushrooms is the variety: white, cremini, oyster, portobello, maitake, reishi, cordyceps. Each offers its own unique blend of health benefits. So in addition to plant-based diversity, I advocate for toadstool diversity!

Pro Tip: Mushrooms
Make sure to cook your mushrooms. Several types contain a substance called agaritine, which is potentially carcinogenic but significantly reduced by cooking.

Seaweed deserves a little more respect. It's not a weed, it's a vegetable. It just so happens to come from the ocean. And what's cool is if we're talking about plant-based diversity, seaweed is a fantastic way to add it because, not only is it high in fiber, but it actually has several unique types of fiber that you won't find in terrestrial plants—ulvans, xylans, agars. Naturally, these are prebiotic fibers. Brown algae, such as kelp or wakame, contain a unique compound called fucoxanthin that helps reduce the accumulation of fats, promotes weight loss, improves insulin sensitivity, and improves blood lipid profiles. Sea veggies are also an excellent source of iodine for thyroid health and vitamin B_{12}.

Since sea veggies and algae aren't a traditional part of the American diet, you may be at a loss for where to start with them. No worries. Let's do a quick little run-through of some options and how to incorporate them.

- **Nori:** These are the crisp sheets that can be softened to make sushi rolls. They're a lightweight, nutritious snack as is, but can also be broken into "flakes" and sprinkled on your salad for some added crunch.
- **Kelp/Kombu:** Generally sold in dried strips and "meaty" versions, kelp adds a nice umami flavor to savory soups, like the Biome Broth (page 249) you'll find in Chapter 10, "The Fiber Fueled 4 Weeks." The Japanese even drink kombu tea.
- **Wakame:** A delicate, lightly sweet seaweed that makes a nice addition to miso soup, or combine it with crunchy veggies like cucumber to make a delicious seaweed salad.
- **Spirulina:** A nutrient-dense blue-green algae found in powder or tablet form that's very high in iron, calcium, protein, B vitamins, and chlorophyll. Sprinkle it into your smoothies and enjoy its deep color.

Public service announcement: Make sure your F GOALS foods are organic!

F GOALS plants are thin-skinned foods. There's no rind or skin to peel away, with the exception of onions and garlic. So any chemical that's sprayed on it is a part of it, and you can't guarantee that you can wash it off. In a prospective cohort study of more than sixty-eight thousand French volunteers, people who ate organic food had a lower overall risk of cancer, non-Hodgkin's lymphoma, and postmenopausal breast cancer. More studies are sure to come, but when considering the addition of industrial chemicals to our food, I think our base position should be one of protection—we should assume that pesticides are poison until proven otherwise.

Adding F GOALS to your daily routine

Okay, so we have our list of foundational foods and now it's time to shift our eating. Be conscious of the fiber and FODMAP content on the F GOALS list. It's no coincidence that these are high-fiber, high FODMAP foods. As we've discussed, FODMAPs aren't the enemy, they're our friend. But whenever we're adding in fiber and FODMAPs, we want to go low and slow to grow—that's the motto.

To view the 60⁺ scientific references cited in this chapter, please visit me online at www.theplantfedgut.com/research/.

PART III
THE FIBER FUELED PLAN

9

Fiber Fueled 365: The Lifestyle

Building healthy habits that lead to
effortless fitness and thriving

We've finally arrived! I'm excited to share the Fiber Fueled 4 Weeks plan with you. But first, let me say that *Fiber Fueled* is not a diet. It's a lifestyle. It is a transformation into the life you deserve, where you restore your health and feel amazing and confident. Take a moment, put this book down, and think about how that transformation looks for you.

It's a beautiful picture, isn't it? Hippocrates, the founder of Western medicine, gave us the adage, "Let your food be your medicine, and your medicine be your food." This idea is central to the *Fiber Fueled* program, but just as important are the healthy lifestyle habits. We'll talk about these later in this chapter: sleep, exercise, time with loved ones, time with yourself, and more. These can be your medicine, too.

When you build the "right routine" then healing just happens. You're living a life that heals, restores, and strengthens you. And it's effortless. But to get there, we have to get into the right frame of mind.

It all starts with a "health mindset"

We are not born with skills that are forever locked in place, incapable of being modified. No one is born to be a professional singer or basketball player, as much as it may seem like that sometimes (hi, Beyoncé and LeBron)—we all have the ability to grow and get better no matter who we are. Rather than believing, "I can't do that," if you apply yourself and get really invested in working toward your goal, you can and will develop new skills and change your life. It's called having a "growth mindset."

The growth mindset is not about who we are but what we are capable of becoming. You are capable of change. The idea of a "growth mindset" was first introduced in Dr. Carol Dweck's book *Mindset: The New Psychology of Success*. It allows you to acknowledge that you have strengths and weaknesses, but that you should celebrate weaknesses as opportunities for growth. With our growth mindset, we choose not to overly emphasize "success" or "skill" or "perfection." We honor effort, learning, and persistence.

My wife and I have been talking about this "growth mindset" since our first child was born. We wanted to create values in our family that embraced perseverance and hard work, not for winning, but for setting a goal to see what you're capable of and what you can make yourself do. We feel strongly that it's a healthy outlook for life.

So I had this awareness already spun into my soul, and when I became motivated to do better with my own health, I started to apply the same concept. I developed a health mindset. I wasn't interested in the pressure of a rigid plan to eat healthy, and I didn't want to go through a painful process of denying myself food through dieting. I wasn't down for shaming and blaming myself for my unhealthy ways or love for fast food. It was time to move forward, but on my own terms.

It wasn't always easy for me and I know it won't always be easy for you. Let me be honest. I loved my old diet. I didn't love the way it made me feel, but for about three minutes, it was blissful to dig into a

Philly cheesesteak or a chili cheese hot dog. I literally was drinking a two-liter bottle of soda almost every day, trying to compensate for the hangover I had after each meal with caffeine. I probably should have been sponsored by Red Bull because they were a regular part of my life; sometimes I had two or three in the same day. And it never hit me that maybe, just maybe, it was my lifestyle that was making me feel like crap and also the reason I couldn't lose weight, even though I was lifting weights for forty-five minutes, then jumping on the treadmill for a 5K or 10K or diving into the pool for a hundred laps.

I wanted to get back to having a healthy relationship with my food in the quest to better myself. I decided to embrace my own starting point and orient my choices toward better health. Every meal became an opportunity to do a little better. And when I slipped up, no worries. I'd try to do better next time. I enjoyed the challenge of seeing what I could do to take care of myself, and the opportunity to learn and grow from it.

It started with little changes. Saying yes to Brussels sprouts. Subbing in a glass of water or kombucha for Coca-Cola Classic or Diet Mountain Dew. Making a delicious smoothie at home rather than stopping at Hardee's to grab a chili cheese dog and burger. No late-night snacks. Dropping the artificial sweeteners and creamer from my coffee. Skipping the french fries sometimes for a side salad to get some green stuff on my plate. I didn't feel deprived or obligated. I was making the choice, and I was choosing better health.

One of the most exciting things I learned on my personal journey is that as I started to make these changes, I found my taste buds came along for the ride. Food that didn't seem appealing to me at first slowly became what I craved. You know that feeling when you return home after travel and you find yourself craving your favorite local meal? For me back in the day that was Jersey Mike's for a cheesesteak or Five Guys for a burger and fries. One day I got home and noticed I was dying for something else—my first stop was to my local salad joint where I grabbed a salad and a kombucha. Look, even to me it still seems weird to say that. I never thought I would crave a salad. But when this started happening to me, I knew something had changed.

The ultimate test came after I'd cleaned up my diet for a few years. I was in medical practice and I had the worst week ever. I was in the hospital by five in the morning every day, and from the moment I walked in the door, I was flying by the seat of my pants trying to get my work done. New consults kept coming in and the number of sick patients I was caring for kept increasing to the point where I was literally running between patients in order to see them all. Plenty of nights I would get stuck in the hospital after hours. Not like, "Hey, I got done at seven-thirty last night." No, this was more like I was lucky if I'd get home by 10:00 p.m. Most nights it would be even later. And it's hard to describe what it does to your morale when you work like that; you hate your job, you hate yourself for taking the job, but what you hate the most is that you haven't seen your wife or newborn daughter awake all week. You get home and they're asleep, then you sneak out in the morning before they get up.

So when the week from hell was over, I said to myself, "You know what . . . you deserve to treat yourself." At this point I was no longer eating red meat. I hadn't had a steak in nearly two years. But once upon a time, when I was chief resident at Northwestern in Chicago, good gracious did I love me a rib eye. So I decided to treat myself to what used to be one of my favorite steak houses. I sat at the bar and ordered a rib eye. Medium rare—that's the way I always liked it.

When the steak came out, though, I didn't start salivating when I smelled it. In fact, something smelled off. And when I took a bite, I knew something definitely was off. It didn't taste the way I remembered. It's not that I felt guilty; heck, I felt like I deserved this reward. It wasn't an ethical thing. I was hungry and I was treating myself. I finished two bites and realized I just didn't want it. I covered it up with my napkin and asked for the bill. I paid the bill and got out of there as quickly as possible before they could question why I didn't like it.

There was nothing wrong with the steak itself. The only thing that had changed were my taste buds. I haven't had a steak since. I have no desire to when it comes to flavor. I had transformed my diet and developed the principles you find in this book by using them in my own life first. I was as happy as I'd ever been, and I wasn't restricting my food intake at all. If I was hungry, I would eat. But I could tell that things had changed for me.

One day I jumped on the scale at work, the same one we use to weigh our patients at each office visit. I'd been between 235 and 240 back in the day, but it'd been years since I actually weighed myself. And as I slid the weights on the scale to find that balance, a smile came across my face. I was down to 190, which is what I weighed in college. Behold the power of plants! And small choices!

Small choices yield huge results, especially as you start to develop more consistency in those small choices. But here's the thing: It's not meant to be a burden. It's about empowering you with a health mindset as your compass toward a better life. It's not about absolutes or being perfect. It's not meant to make you feel guilty when you grab the fries and soda. Absolutely not. Adopting a health mindset means finding the positives and celebrating progress rather than flogging ourselves for moments of weakness or imperfection. We all have those moments—myself included! But don't let them make you give up.

If your taste buds aren't quite there yet, don't worry. You'll get there just like I did. As your microbiome changes, so will your taste buds. The changes that you make to your diet over time will change the core of your microbiome—remember how adaptable it is?—and ultimately your taste will evolve with it. Trust me; these foods that you don't think you have a taste for now are going to be your new obsession!

Even better news is that you don't have to wait for your microbiome to shift by torturing yourself or pretending you need to eat food that you don't like. Remember, you have three hundred thousand edible plants to choose from! It's not just diversity of plants, either—there's diversity of flavors, too. All herbs and spices are plants and most flavors from around the world are inspired by plants, so Mexican, Italian, Greek, Thai, Japanese, Chinese, Vietnamese, Ethiopian, and more are all fair game. There are so many ways to eat plants: soups, salads, smoothies, sandwiches, stews, and more. Those are just the S's. We haven't even talked about noodles, tacos, pita wraps, rice bowls . . . the list goes on.

We each have our own starting point. And while the tools in this book can help everyone on their journey, the end point will look different for each person. What I'm about is progress. According to the U.S. Department of Agriculture, the average American gets just 11 percent of their calories from whole grains, beans, fruits, vegetables, seeds, and nuts. That's *average*. In other words, if you're reading this book and you get 5 percent of your calories from plants, you're actually pretty darn close to the average. And you have the most room to benefit from small changes. If you move that needle from 5 to 30 percent, you can improve your health. Then watch those small changes add up.

Strive for 90 percent

I don't want you to feel burdened by the lifestyle changes I'm suggesting—I want you to feel excited about the possibility you have for growth! But it's good to have a goal. Otherwise you may just be wandering around aimlessly eating blueberries and hoping for the best. So let's strive toward becoming 90 percent plant-based. Not necessarily today, but that's our big-picture goal. Why 90 percent? Well, this is what we see in the Blue Zones population—they are 90 percent plant-based, so we know it's a diet that will give you enormous health benefits. Plus, having a little leniency helps avoid the pressure of being "perfect." That 10 percent is your sandbox. You get to make what you want of it. Whatever your vice, it can fit into your 10 percent flex account so you don't have to feel guilty about it.

Let's be clear on what constitutes 90 percent here. I'm talking about whole plant foods. Things you can actually grow in soil. Things that don't come in boxes or special packages. Things that don't have ingredient lists because there's only one ingredient—a plant. Everything else falls outside the 90 percent—processed plant foods, oil, meat, and dairy. There are plenty of vegans who should clean up their diet. Veganism is not automatically a healthy diet just because you've eliminated animal products. There are lots of unhealthy processed plant foods out there, and lots of unhealthy vegans.

Let's talk about oil, folks!

You're all wondering, "What's the deal with oil?" so here it is. . . . Oil is a processed food. By definition, it is high-calorie, low-nutrient. A pound of greens has 100 calories. A pound of oil has over 4,000! Olive oil is healthier than the alternative oils, and so when you opt for oil I'd generally recommend extra-virgin olive oil. But do you want to guess how many grams of fiber there are in olive oil? Zero. Same is true for all oil varietals. Zero grams of fiber, no matter which type or amount. We should not be striving to get more oil in our life, so that's why it's part of our 10 percent flex account.

Make no mistake about it, I'm not encouraging you to stop at 90 percent. That would be inconsistent with our health mindset. I honestly believe that you're going to feel so good as you incorporate more fresh plants into your diet that you're going to want more and more, and that's going to drive you closer to 100 percent. How do I know this? Because that's what happened with me. I came to a point where I was close but not quite there, and I decided to give up the last few pieces. I have to tell you, I was surprised by how much of a difference giving up even that last small piece was. Why have something hold you back? But at the end of the day, no matter who you are and what your matter of perspective is, this is about challenging yourself to improve. This is about personal growth toward a more plant-centered diet. How exactly that's going to look is personalized and your choice. But whether you're 15 percent or 95 percent, if you're moving in the right direction, then I am your biggest cheerleader and with you 100 percent. Let's do it together and share our common philosophy.

When healthy habits form, effortless fitness ensues

If I asked you to close your eyes and envision what medicine looks like, what would you come up with? Is it a pill? A doctor wearing a white coat and reaching out with a stethoscope? Do you see yourself lying in a hospital bed, hooked up to an IV and a nurse checking your vital signs?

What if medicine could be you, right now . . . living, breathing, in the flesh. Not an intervention by our reactive health care system, but instead just you living your routine daily life.

It's time for us to redefine health care and acknowledge that health during our lifetime is the sum of all of the small choices we make minute by minute, day by day. One choice, whether good or bad, makes little to no difference in the grand scheme of things. People don't drop dead from having one cigarette. But if you create consistency, a pattern, then you are amplifying that choice over the course of time.

We are creatures of habit. There's just no getting away from that. That can be problematic when we form bad habits that take a poor choice and amplify it. But the flip side is that we can acknowledge the power in our habits to amplify our choices, and use it to our advantage by being intentional in creating healthy habits.

It is these healthy habits that can allow us to just live our routine lives and yet be promoting health and fitness. It becomes effortless because it's just our routine, but when our routine promotes health it's so much more powerful than any pill a doctor could give you. The body is designed to heal if we can just get out of its way.

In the coming pages you will find the lifestyle elements that contribute to a healthy gut. Think of each of these as a small opportunity around which to build a healthy habit. Remember, small changes yield big results, and when we make them our habits, effortless fitness ensues. Here are the pillars of a *Fiber Fueled* life:

Diversity of plants is the number one predictor of a healthy gut microbiota

At this point, you probably don't need me to explain why the Golden Rule of plant-based diversity matters. You've heard it throughout this book. This is our anthem. Our core philosophy. We no longer need a laundry list of food rules, we only need to remember to eat a diversity of plants. When you walk into the supermarket, remember: "Diversity of plants." When you're at the salad bar, trying to figure out what to add, remember: "Diversity of plants." "Diversity of plants" should cross your mind whenever you're thinking about what to eat. It will help you in your quest to maximize plant-based diversity.

And remember: Plant-based diversity is a celebration of nature's abundance. You get to taste and enjoy all the flavors, all the textures. Herbs and spices abound. Gone are the days of dietary restriction and lists of "approved" foods. Is it a plant? Okay, cool, we're good. We should be striving to include at least thirty different plants per week. But truly, if you're on a mission to maximize diversity with each meal, you're going to *crush* that goal.

What's better—raw or cooked?

New research indicates that the same plant will have different effects on the gut microbiome in raw and cooked forms. Cooking alters the carbohydrates, like fiber, and many of the chemicals in the plants. The result is a different effect on microbial growth, the genetic makeup of the microbiome, and the types of postbiotics generated. While we can't say that one is necessarily better, we can say that they're different. Here's a pro tip: If you're cooking your food, make sure to nibble on some of the raw ingredients to get their unique benefits and add even more plant-based diversity to your meal.

Strive toward gut fitness by exercising your gut

There are some of you who will struggle with this process more than others. As we discussed in Chapter 5, you may need the help of a doctor to make sure there's no constipation, food allergy, celiac disease, or alternative explanation for your issues. If you've ruled out everything except food sensitivity, then we need to identify the strengths and weaknesses within your gut. We all have them! Rather than looking at food as black and white—either you tolerate or you don't—we should instead be looking at the shades of gray. There's a certain amount you can tolerate and that's entirely personal and determined by your individual gut microbiota.

As part of the Fiber Fueled 4 Weeks (see Chapter 10), I've labeled the moderate- and high-FODMAP ingredients and even offered substitutions. This way, if you have a meal and then develop digestive distress, it gives you an idea of which ingredient may have been problematic. A food diary can help you keep notes and potentially identify triggers. Among the FODMAPs, there may be specific categories that cause more trouble for you than others—fructose, fructans, galactans, or polyols. It could be lactose if you're consuming dairy as well, although I would eliminate dairy if you're having ongoing digestive issues.

If you identify which FODMAPs cause the most trouble, then you know which ones you need to ease into. Plan to go back to the same recipe in the future and make low FODMAP substitutions and see if it's a better experience for you. But if it remains a mystery and you just don't seem to be making progress, even after going through the Fiber Fueled 4 Weeks, then you may need to work with a registered dietitian to do a formal FODMAP elimination and reintroduction. This is a lengthy and fairly complex process, and it takes more than twenty-eight days to complete. But if you need to do it, make sure you do it right under the guidance of a qualified professional.

F GOALS: The foundation on which plant-based diversity is built

In Chapter 8 we explored the health benefits of our F GOALS foods. These are the gut health superfoods on which we want to build our microbiome, and the starting point or core diet. Plant-based diversity remains the mission, and F GOALS are the fundamental foods in that mission. In them, you'll find all the good stuff: SCFA-producing fiber, vitamins, minerals, microbes, and unique phytochemicals like sulfora-phane. I'm challenging you to step your game up and have something from this list every day.

Is a little meat and dairy okay?

We discussed in Chapter 2 that there are healthy and unhealthy proteins and fats. Plants and animal products clearly have different effects on the gut microbiota and on health outcomes. Whether you choose to include animal products in your diet is ultimately your choice, but the bottom line from my perspective is that it doesn't improve your health. I personally have opted to eliminate animal products from my diet and feel great in doing so. But I also can't say that you're "unhealthy" if you continue to consume a small amount. By small, I mean radically different than the 220 pounds of meat and 30 pounds of cheese that the average American is currently consuming. Again, I believe in being at least 90 percent plant-based. What you do with that last 10 percent is up to you, but I am challenging you to continue your health mindset, to never accept stagnation, and to strive toward better health.

Some people may wonder: Are grass-fed hormone- and antibiotic-free animal products good for your health? Well, yes compared to antibiotic-laden, hormone-infused, GMO-fed animal meats, but that's like saying chewing tobacco is healthier than smoking a cigarette. It doesn't mean it's actually good for you— it's just relatively better. I'd encourage you to spend some time deciding where you stand.

Should the environmental impact or ethics of our food choices be considered? I believe we all have a responsibility to educate ourselves and come to our own conclusions. Remember, we don't just have a microbiome in our guts; the soil does, the plants do, and animals do, too. The twentieth and twenty-first centuries haven't been very kind to any of them, which is a result of human activity.

If you choose to taper down your animal products, one approach is an elimination progression, moving up the chain to higher-quality substitutions over the course of time:

Eliminate Beef > Pork > Chicken > Eggs > Salmon and then land on Tofu and Beans

F GOALS

F: Fruit (spotlight on berries) & Fermented
G: Greens & Grains

O: Omega-3 Super Seeds

A: Aromatics (onions, garlic)

L: Legumes

S: Sulforaphane (broccoli sprouts and other cruciferous veggies)

In Chapter 8 we learned a few tricks to get the most from our F GOALS foods. Mushrooms should be cooked, while aromatics and cruciferous vegetables are generally best enjoyed raw. Aromatics and cruciferous veggies have enzymes that need to be activated to maximize the health benefits, so we can use the CHOP then STOP trick to bring out those phytochemicals. When it comes to super seeds, remember: flax for lignans, chia for fiber, hemp for protein. Or why not all three in a morning smoothie? And don't be shy about adding greens at every single meal, even if it's just a handful that you eat raw. They are maximum nutrients with minimum calories. Put your foot down on the accelerator and go all out on them.

Don't overlook the importance of hydration

For years I would roll out of bed and walk like a zombie to the coffeepot. I'd spend the next couple of hours trying to feel alive, attempting to slap the fatigue out of my face with caffeine. At some point I'd cross that line and feel awake, but then also strangely strung out and jittery from too much caffeine. Why couldn't this be simple?

It can be. It starts with water, the simplest, healthiest, and least expensive beverage on the planet. I'm as guilty of this as anyone, but it's amazing that we pay several dollars to drink a soda or something else that's going to hurt us when restaurants will provide you ice water for free. Frankly, we should be more appreciative of our access to water. It's a requirement for life. At least 60 percent of your body is composed of water. You could go three weeks without food but you wouldn't last more than four days without water. It's vital! And life giving.

Unfortunately our twenty-first-century lifestyle is ignoring this health marvel. For most of us, our most dehydrated time during the day is when we first wake up. We haven't had anything to drink for several hours, and so it's the ideal time to rehydrate our bodies. In the last few years I changed my routine to start with two large glasses of water. It's amazing the difference this little change provides. It turns on my brain, gut, and kidneys and I feel much more awake. I still reach for the coffee, but after I've had my water.

Then, as the morning progresses, I make sure to keep things balanced between coffee and water. There's no more straight coffee. I'm doing both, but favoring more water than coffee. I pay attention to my lips now. When I feel my lips getting a little chapped I'll grab the water bottle.

To optimize hydration, my recommendation is to wake up and have two large glasses of water first thing in the morning like I do. Make sure to drink more water than coffee or other caffeinated product in the morning. Add two glasses of water to each meal. This will help you get up to eight glasses of water per day and help your body function the way it was meant to.

Let's choose refreshments that actually refresh us

It's really not that hard to incorporate healing salves into your beverage selection. Small changes yield massive results when it's your daily routine, and this is one we can easily take advantage of! Here are some great ways to make better beverage selections to amp up your gut health throughout the day:

- **Jazz up your water:** I love a good squeeze of citrus in my water and have more than gotten my money's worth from my juice squeezer. Throw a couple of slices of citrus and some water in a giant mason jar with some ice on a great summer day. Or infuse your water overnight with cucumbers or

watermelon and mint and pamper yourself with spa-worthy
hydration.

- **A little coffee in the morning:** I'm a believer! Coffee contains
polyphenols that act as prebiotics for the microbiota. It's also the
biggest source of antioxidants in the Western diet right now. I'm
trying to change that by spreading the *Fiber Fueled* message, but
in the meantime I don't see a reason to give it up. The problem
with coffee is the junk we throw in it. I converted to straight
black coffee, and I love it. But if you absolutely must add a
sweetener, a little bit of stevia, monk fruit, or erythritol will do
the trick. And creamer? I'd skip the dairy and go with organic soy
milk. I know lots of people who love unsweetened oat milk in
their coffee. I also love spicing up my coffee—cinnamon, ginger,
and turmeric is a fave combo. If I'm dragging and need an extra
kick, I'll drop some maca and ashwagandha in there. These are
adaptogenic superfoods derived from roots that combat fatigue
and stress. If I'm adding spices, I'm usually adding some organic
soy milk and sweetener as well to soften the flavors. But keep your
coffee to two cups max. Also remember to pound the water
before, during, and after coffee consumption. Finally, if you have
a diarrhea-related issue, such as irritable bowel, coffee may
aggravate your symptoms.

A note on caffeine

I generally am not opposed to caffeine. Okay, fine, I'll admit—I
love it. Couldn't have survived internship without it. But some of
you may suffer from caffeine sensitivity, which can exacerbate
digestive issues. There's actually a gene that causes this. If
you're worried about this possibility, I'd consider eliminating all
caffeine for a week and see how you feel.

- **Green tea in the afternoon:** One of my favorite rituals is to have hot green tea an hour or two after lunch. It really invigorates me for the afternoon, and tea has a phytochemical called L-theanine that improves focus. You'll notice the difference compared to coffee. Green tea is also an excellent source of prebiotic polyphenols. My specific recommendation for green tea is organic ceremonial-grade matcha tea. It's rich in antioxidants and offers literally one hundred times more prebiotic polyphenol EGCG than conventional green tea. All you have to do is add hot water, although you can crank the antioxidants even higher with a squeeze of citrus because the vitamin C dramatically improves their absorption, meaning you get even more from the same cup of tea. Speaking of which, try making a matcha cooler by throwing matcha in a mason jar with some ice and a lemon. It's a drink that makes me think of Arnold Palmer, the late great golfer, who loved combining iced tea and lemonade.

- **Smoothies over juice:** I'm not anti-juice. I'm just pro-smoothie. What are you doing when you create the juice? That's right, separating the fiber and then throwing it out. Removing the fiber but keeping the sugar gives me a bad case of processed food déjà vu. Remember, we want to be *Fiber Fueled*. But that said, I've also been preaching "low and slow, that is the motto" when it comes to fiber, and since smoothies are such a beautifully dense heaping of fiber, it may be too much for some of you as you ramp up fiber and FODMAPs. In that case, juice can help to get you the phytonutrients without pushing you too hard on the fiber. But juices shouldn't be piña colada–flavored, they should be at least somewhat bitter. If you're making a fruit juice, you're basically creating a sugar beverage. Fructose in whole fruit is fine, but when you toss the fiber it becomes straight sugar. So when making juice, my recommendation is to use almost exclusively veggies with minimal fruit and embrace the bitter flavor!

- **Easy on the 'booch:** I love kombucha and drink it routinely. I think it can definitely be a part of a healthy lifestyle, but there's a lot of hype that's motivating people to slug down 32 ounces per day and rely on it as their only fermented food. I'd far rather you drink 'booch than soda or other sweetened beverages, but the acidity can erode the enamel on your teeth, so I always dilute it down substantially. Drink it with at least half water. I only drink 4 or so ounces per day, a fraction of a 16-ounce bottle you can buy at the store. But that 4 ounces turns into 8 to 12 for me after I dilute it down.

- **Avoid alcohol:** I know this isn't what some of you want to hear, but if we're building a healthy gut I would recommend avoidance of alcohol. It's clear that binge alcohol consumption causes damage to the gut microbiota, increasing intestinal permeability, and the release of bacterial endotoxin. In other words, alcohol causes dysbiosis. Believe it or not, this is how alcohol causes cirrhosis. You don't have to be an alcoholic, either. Just a single crazy Friday night can damage your gut. Is it possible that these rules don't apply to light drinking, though? Unfortunately, not. Just one drink per day increases your risk of high blood pressure and stroke. Just a half drink per day has been associated with increased risk of cancer. There is strong consensus among the scientific community that alcohol causes cancer. We shouldn't be so surprised, though—alcohol kills bacteria, and in the case of our guts, this can mean it attacks our "good" bugs.

Are the rules different for red wine?

Some experts argue that red wine is good for us because it has the polyphenol resveratrol. It's true that polyphenols in red wine are prebiotic and can increase gut diversity. It's also true that resveratrol in red wine has been linked with heart health, but it wasn't until recently that we discovered the mechanism—once again involving gut bacteria. Resveratrol in red wine decreases TMAO levels by inhibiting the production of TMA by the gut microbiota. TMA is the precursor to TMAO. We know from Chapter 2 that TMAO comes from consumption of meat, eggs, and high-fat dairy and has been implicated in the pathogenesis of heart disease, stroke, Alzheimer's, type 2 diabetes, and chronic kidney disease. Five of the top ten killers. In a country that eats more meat than any other in the world, of course having a way to slow down TMAO production would benefit the heart, but drinking red wine to do it can create alcohol dependence and potentially cirrhosis. Why not just reduce our red meat consumption and eat more plants? Grapes, blueberries, raspberries, mulberries, and even peanuts have resveratrol, but without the risks. That said, if we're going to responsibly enjoy alcohol, the occasional glass of red wine would be the way to do it.

Activate your satiety hormones naturally

We've all been conditioned to focus on the amount of food—whether we're counting calories or macronutrient percentages of whatever. I've heard of diets where people even weigh their food. It can be so complicated! But it doesn't have to be. Let me make this incredibly simple: When you reach for whole plant foods, you can eat WITHOUT RESTRICTION. No exaggeration, you have my green light to eat as much as you want. I'm going to say it again. Eat as much as you want. You'll still lose weight and get all the health benefits.

Here's why this works: Thank the fiber and resistant starch. Whole plant foods are by definition high nutrient, low calorie. There is the requirement to actually chew them; you can't just inhale them. We know that chewing takes time. When we eat a salad, it takes longer than eating a hot dog. As we learned in Chapter 3, fiber and resistant starches produce SCFAs that trigger the release of satiety hormones. By taking our time to chew fiber-rich food, we are allowing our body to use its natural mechanisms to tell us when we've had enough. No need to count calories. Mother Nature is counting them for you. You'll feel full and satisfied, and know that it's been enough. And it will be a meal jam-packed with nutrients and fiber.

For most of human history, our species consumed whole plant foods to the tune of 100 grams of fiber or more per day. This was real food that grew in the dirt. Not fried okra, veggie burgers, processed grains like bread, or nondairy ice cream. When we process our food, we strip away the fiber. We pervert nature's balance and create artificially calorie-dense, fiber-poor foods that encourage overeating. Processed foods are the majority of America's diet. Most of the rest is meat, dairy, eggs, and oil. Calorically dense with a net fiber offering of zero. And then we wonder why we overeat and have an obesity problem and the associated health issues.

If you flip the ratio by following the plan in this book and eat 90 to 100 percent plant-based with diversity of plants, counting calories will not be necessary. You can eat when you're hungry, eat until you're full and satisfied, and you'll still lose weight thanks to being *Fiber Fueled*.

Engage in mindful eating

Go, go, go! That's the American lifestyle these days. I'm as guilty as anyone. I push myself to move faster, do more, and I sometimes skip meals. Let's start by taking a deep breath. There are some things in life that are too important to let the rat race infringe on them. It's unhealthy to inhale your food. The process of digestion starts in your mouth, where mastication breaks up the food and amylase in saliva begins to break down the starches. When we eat too fast, we don't allow our body to catch up with what we're doing, which leads to overeating. We weren't designed to scarf down food and get it over as quickly as possible; we're wired to enjoy our food and allow our body to signal us when it's full.

When I was a kid my Granddaddy would always say, "Small bites, and chew well!" We all need to follow Granddaddy's sage advice by reengaging with our food. Mindful eating is simply getting back to our roots of enjoying our food. It's having the manners that your grandparents taught you when you were a kid. Here's how you do it:

- **Sit down at an actual table.** No eating in the car or while you walk. Put your food on a plate or in a bowl. Don't eat out of a container.
- **Turn off your cell phone.** Put down your laptop. Shut off the TV. No electronics during this sacred time.
- **Spend a moment observing your food before you start.** Celebrate nature's bounty—the looks, the smells. It's beautiful.
- **Take a moment to taste your food.** It doesn't have to be with every bite, but you should routinely take moments to pause.
- **Chew your food!** Not one or two chomps. I'm talking twenty-five or more bites. Set your fork down while you chew.
- **Observe the Japanese tradition of *hara hachi bu*.** As described in *The Blue Zones*, this means eating until you're 80 percent full and then stopping. By doing this, you're giving your body a chance to catch up so that you're just right and not overshooting.
- **Enjoy meals with other people when you can.** The Europeans have mastered this and we Americans are struggling. We should be taking our time and enjoying each other's company while we eat, not sprinting to inhale our food so we can get back to work.
- **Schedule your mealtimes.** Maintain a regular schedule that taps into your circadian rhythm. An early dinnertime is key. I'll talk more about this in the next section.

- **Avoid toxic hunger.** Eating as a reaction to hunger or to emotion is an unhealthy practice. You're far more likely to reach for unhealthy "comfort" foods than nourishing, healthy foods. If you feel hunger coming on, don't wait until it's turned you into a carb-starved monster. This is where a piece of fruit or a handful of nuts can do the trick to hold you over until your next scheduled mealtime.

It's not just what you eat but *when* you eat that matters . . .

Our body has a natural biorhythm that we call our circadian rhythm. This is an endogenous, entrainable oscillation of about twenty-four hours that's a part of all life throughout our planet—other animals, plants, fungi. They all have this. Our gut microbes are no exception! When you disrupt your natural rhythm you are also perturbing your microbes. For example, jet lag actually induces dysbiosis in the gut microbes, which is why you feel like trash when flying internationally. And don't get me started on the shared cultural nightmare that is daylight saving time. If you are a shift worker, you probably also know this feeling well. Shift workers are at increased risk for hypertension, hyperlipidemia, obesity, and type 2 diabetes because of what a disrupted circadian rhythm does to the gut microbiome.

Our gut microbes thrive on consistency that's anchored into these twenty-four-hour oscillations, and that means timely meals. For example, you can eat literally the exact same food but at different times in the day and have a different effect on your blood sugar. We are most insulin sensitive in the morning and most insulin resistant in the evening. To optimize our eating patterns, we want to anchor our eating around the times that we need our fuel, and then allow our gut to rest for a period of time. This approach is called time-restricted eating, or TRE. Some call it intermittent fasting, but this isn't intermittent. It's a lifestyle that you sustain day to day.

To properly do TRE, you have to do two things. First, you create time boundaries so there's a period of food consumption and a period of sustained bowel rest. My recommendation is to rest your gut for at least thirteen consecutive hours, which means restricting your eating hours to eleven or less.

Second, you need to synchronize your eating pattern with your circadian biology. This is the part that many people are overlooking. It's not just any thirteen hours. Do you need to have a big meal in the evening or have a snack at 10:00 p.m.? Of course not. TRE is not meant to be first meal at 11:00 a.m. and last meal at 10:00 p.m. That's a whacked-out biorhythm. To get things properly aligned, you should eat dinner early in the evening and then it's a hard line—no food after dinner! Just water. It's also important to create a space of at least two if not three hours between when you stop eating and your bedtime. The earlier the better on dinner.

Does coffee break the fast?

Yes and no. Fasting benefits the gut microbes because they get a break to reset, and anything but water interrupts that. But the fat-burning metabolic benefits continue if you drink coffee and avoid solid food. I personally have had great success with twelve hours of strict water fasting followed by coffee and delaying my first solid food for a few more hours in the morning.

On the topic of optimizing our biorhythm, let's talk about meal size. We tend to gorge ourselves at dinner, but it doesn't really make sense. We don't need a massive dinner when we should be winding down for sleep shortly after. On the flip side, we've been overlooking lunch. Midday is when we need energy the most. So let's invest a little more into a nice, satisfying lunch.

Supplements are meant to supplement diet and lifestyle, not replace them

As we discussed in Chapter 7, you can't overcome a bad diet or unhealthy lifestyle with supplements. We also see a lot of hype around supplements in the absence of science. Many of the most popular supplements on the market have little to no research to actually support them. They can be a waste of your money or, worse yet, they can harm you because they're not different from taking a medication. At least with medicine we know what the risks are. If you take five or more supplements because they're "natural," I can assure you that no one knows what they are doing in combination.

But I do believe there's a role for supplements when properly used. They allow us to optimize our diet. As we discussed in Chapter 7, I'm a believer in prebiotics and in some cases probiotics. There are three supplements that I generally recommend to address some of the challenges in our twenty-first-century life: vitamin B_{12}, vitamin D, and an algae-based omega-3 supplement. It's best to discuss these with your doctor to determine if they make sense for you and, if so, what dosage you should take.

Sleep is powerfully restorative

It's actually incredible the way your body heals when you just allow it to rest. You can think of time-restricted eating as rest for your gut. But sleep is rest for the entire body, including the gut. When we deprive ourselves of sleep, we feel the effects in the microbiome as it shifts toward a profile promoting obesity. No wonder we feel so crummy after a poor night's rest. Insufficient sleep is associated with increased appetite, weight gain, increased risk of heart disease/stroke/diabetes, impaired immunity, depression, poor concentration/productivity/work performance, and even poor athletic performance. Sleep is free and it powerfully promotes better health, including in your microbes.

It's important not only that we get enough sleep, but also that it's anchored to our circadian biology. The circadian rhythm in sleep and wakefulness is primarily synchronized to the rise and fall of the sun. When you get up in the morning, make it a point to expose yourself to natural sunlight. Even a short walk outside can work wonders. On the flip side, we need to wind down when the sun goes down at night. Ideally, we should stop using electronics during this time because the bright light impairs melatonin release. We should also strive toward an earlier bedtime. In the words of Ben Franklin, "Early to bed and early to rise makes a man healthy, wealthy and wise."

Time to reconnect with nature

Speaking of seeing the sun, think of how much life has changed for us humans in the last few hundred years. We went from predominantly outdoor creatures to the sterile, bleached interior of our homes and offices. Seems safer, but is it? We've certainly drifted away from nature. We've seen in this book that living creatures either have a microbiota or are a part of the microbiota. Microbes are a fundamental part of life on Earth. So what happens when we surround ourselves with lifeless physical structures (our homes) that we spray with chemicals? Unlike the lush habitats in nature, our man-made structures are a microbial badland that fails to contribute to your microbial diversity. No surprise, moving from a rural environment to the city has been associated with the loss of beneficial microbes and an increase in dangerous genes.

Conceptually this goes back to the hygiene hypothesis discussed in Chapter 1. Exposure to the outdoors early in life has been shown to improve immune function. Adults who exercise outdoors have more diverse microbiomes. Gardening improves mood, lowers stress, increases life satisfaction, and even promotes weight loss. Not to mention that growing your own veggies has been shown to make you enjoy eating them even more! We've even found that barefoot contact with the earth can improve mood, boost creativity, and give you more restful sleep.

The point is we need to look for opportunities to get outdoors.

Don't run on the treadmill when you could actually run outside. Don't buy your plants when you could grow them. Don't read this book on the couch when you could throw down a blanket and take off your shoes outside. And since we will continue to live indoors, let's make the most of it and decorate our homes and offices with potted plants. Making time to trade microbes with nature is a necessary and wildly underrated contributor to human health. Every single one of us should have an outdoor hobby for every season of the year.

Regular exercise contributes to gut health

I find it amazing the way that fitness contributes to gut fitness. Our movement pattern, whether active or sluggish, ultimately has an effect on our microbes. In mice we see exercise induce dramatic changes in the gut microbiota, with more SCFA producers and improved intestinal integrity. Believe it or not, there was a 40 percent increase in healthy microbes with exercise. Similarly, in adult humans we see increased SCFA-producing gut microbes with regular exercise. The effect is lost when you stop moving.

The fact that SCFA-producing microbes are generated through exercise says a lot. Mother Nature rewards us for good behavior, and the currency is SCFAs. Whether it's healthy eating or exercise, they share a common pathway that leads to health benefit. Once again, all signs point toward the relevance of SCFAs in human health. This explains why a healthy diet and exercise are individually great but in combination you get a synergistic effect.

Take a short fifteen- to thirty-minute walk after dinner, for example. Research shows us that it helps mobilize and empty your stomach, which helps digestion and reduces the likelihood of having acid reflux. A short walk stabilizes blood sugar and reduces triglycerides, contributing to a lower risk of coronary heart disease. Fat is burned and weight is lost. Your immune system gets stronger and risk of infection declines. Your energy levels and mood are lifted up. A walk outside even unlocks the creative part of your brain. All of this from just having a healthy routine that involves a walk after dinner. So easy!

Make no mistake—you can't exercise your way out of a bad diet. I've proven that firsthand. The benefits of exercise and plant-based eating go hand in hand. If exercise is not currently a part of your life-style, try walking at least thirty minutes three times a week. But if you only have ten minutes, start there. You can work to increase your time. When you exercise, it's going to hurt a little in the beginning, but it'll get better as you get stronger. Just like when you exercise your gut.

We need human connection to thrive

The highest form of torture is isolation, removing a person from other humans. We are by definition social creatures; it's a part of our biol-ogy. We're living in the era of "social media," yet are more isolated than ever. Social media is not only antisocial; it's bad for our mental health and may be bad for our gut.

Life and microbes are meant to be shared with others. Believe it or not, each one of us has a unique "bacterial cloud" that follows us around. We're each emitting about a million particles into our envi-ronment per hour. Close proximity to others has the potential for sharing among our bacterial cloud. Studies show that you're likely to share microbiome similarities with the people you live with. These relationships have even been shown to impact our genetic expression. Even having our furry friends—dogs and cats—can contribute to mi-crobiome health and protect us from disease. Our environment and the people we surround ourselves with allow a microbial exchange that keeps us alive and thriving. In a hypersterile world, I celebrate the microbes that some call germs or dirty.

We need to get back to the basics of spending time with real peo-ple: shaking hands, giving high fives, looking someone in the eye when they're talking. It's time to put down the phone and get back to how we're wired—for human connection.

Stress management is key

Stress impacts the gut. In fact, stress alone can create alterations in the gut microbiota and an increase in intestinal permeability leading to dysbiosis. This is why you can drink your green smoothie, eat your plants, go to the gym, and get a good night's rest, but if your heart and head aren't at peace then neither are your microbes. Many of the worst digestive issues that I see in my clinic are in the victims of abuse or those recovering from an eating disorder.

The good news is that the opposite is also true. Stress-reducing practices, such as meditation, are actually good for your gut. Take away the stress and suddenly the gut microbiota increase production of SCFAs and anti-inflammatory metabolites. All signs point to the importance of self-care and having a stress management practice. Some would call this mindfulness.

It can be simple. Just five minutes at least once a day in a quiet space. Settle into a comfortable position, loosen your clothes. This is your time, but you're going to dedicate it to the positive things in your life. There are four steps. First, think of something you're grateful for. Focus on a positive thing that's happened to you. Second, think of someone you love. Take a moment to appreciate the positive role they have in your life. Third, clarify your intention. You're drawing a map to where you want to go. What do you want to happen in your life? This can be anything—an emotion, behavior, or goal. Make sure it's positive and something immediately applicable in the short term. Last but not least, release your mind, focus on your breathing, and allow thoughts to naturally enter your mind. End with a few deep breaths and focus your eyes softly.

To view the 45+ scientific references cited in this chapter, please visit me online at www.theplantfedgut.com/research/.

10

The Fiber Fueled 4 Weeks

Become a plant-based rock star

In my mind I imagine we're sitting across from each other at a coffee shop, not my office—this isn't a medical visit. We're talking about all the big things: life, health, family. Our values. To me, taking care of our health is crucial to all aspects of our life. And I hope I've convinced you to believe the same. The *Fiber Fueled* four-week plan is the start of the new you—it lets you lead your life with energy, vitality, and confidence, while you protect your body from disease.

Obviously making the transition to a plant-based diet has some challenges. We're up against habits, cravings, and even addiction to our meat, dairy, sugar, fat, and processed grains. Quitting these foods can literally cause withdrawal symptoms. Cravings will certainly happen. It's going to take some effort to change old habits, believe me, I know.

But just know that we're all in this together. You are not alone. And I will give you the tools you need to make this shift. This program was designed for my own patients, as a way to optimize the gut, eliminate cravings, strengthen the immune system, improve energy levels, and resolve digestive issues. If this can work for them, it can work for you, too. In just twenty-eight days you'll take back your health, break the chains of food addiction, amplify your plant diversity, build a strategy for food sensitivity, and reemerge as the fitter, healthier, and happier person you deserve to be. Are you ready for it? Okay, let's get started!

What's in the Fiber Fueled 4 Weeks

In the coming pages you'll find more than sixty-five mouthwatering, plant-based recipes organized into a twenty-eight-day calendar for you. I'm sure the suspense is killing you, so if you want to flip ahead and check out a couple of them, I don't blame you! Super Seedy Breakfast Porridge (page 223) with a Matcha Latte (page 275) . . . The Daily Salad (page 229) with Supercharged Roasted Roots (page 231) and Oil-Free Orange Dressing (page 230) . . . Creamy polenta with quick lentil ragu (Plant-Powered Polenta Ragu, page 235) . . . Folks, that's just Day 1.

You are going to have an incredible month filled with delicious food thanks to my friend Alexandra Caspero. Alex is a registered dietitian and recipe developer who shares my food philosophy. We both believe that plant foods are delicious, healthy, and to be enjoyed in abundance. So we developed the Fiber Fueled 4 Weeks together to manifest the teachings of this book but also to offer an individualized experience. We recognize that there is no "one size fits all."

To that end, for each of the twenty-eight days you'll find three recipes: breakfast, lunch, and dinner—but of course! Those are spelled out on a daily basis for you. But then we also have the weekly drink, snack, and dessert recipes. We give you a few of those each week to enhance your experience as you deem fit. They could be daily, or you may not use them at all: It's whatever works best for you.

One of our priorities in the Fiber Fueled 4 Weeks was to make this as easy as possible for you. Let's be honest, doing a twenty-eight-day plan in any book isn't easy. We know that going in. Easy would be picking up fast food on the way home from a long day's work. Instead, you're going to be cooking food. You're going to be picking up groceries. Lots of them, because that's what plant-based diversity is about. But in developing our Fiber Fueled 4 Weeks, we really wanted to control what we could and ease your burden.

So we intentionally pushed for recipes that are reasonably simple while still emphasizing diversity of plants. We're also providing you with additional resources to make this easier for you. Every week there is a shopping list. It's here in this book, but if you'd like it in a printable version so that you can easily carry it into the market, email me at shoppinglist@theplantfedgut.com and I'll be happy to share that with you.

We've also built in a cooking day once a week. We suggest you pick one day where you'll spend a few hours prepping meals for the week. We have it listed as Sunday, because that's what most of you will do. But if a different day is better for you, feel free to switch it up. Prep day will allow you to have several things premade and ready to go, paying dividends later in the week when you need to throw something together in two seconds.

We also have several days where you'll reuse a recipe, most of the time with a new spin on the second go-round. For example, you'll prep the Biome Broth (page 249) (our take on plant-based bone broth) for Week 1, then use it for Wild Biome Super Soup (page 232) on Day 2, and even use it to build a Miso, Mushroom, and Soba Bowl (page 271) in Week 2. Or there's the Tempeh Tacos (page 236) on Day 2 followed by the Tempeh Taco Salad (page 237) with Creamy Cilantro Sauce (page 237) on Day 4. All this talk is making you hungry, isn't it?

Finally, this plan isn't about tough love and testing your persistence. This plan is the philosophy in this book: progress over perfection, plants in abundance, slow and low with fiber and FODMAPs, training the gut and working toward 90 percent or more plant-based. With that in mind, we encourage you to modify it based upon your individual needs. If you need to add meat on top, so be it. Progress over perfection. If you aren't excited about a recipe and you want to redo one of the ones from earlier in the week, just do it. And if you come home from work and don't have time to cook, don't worry because we have included Quick-Fix recipes (see pages 220, 256, 283, and 317) that you can turn to if you're not in the mood to cook. Basically, we want you to march your way through this plan and emerge on the other side as a healthier version of yourself, and do it on your terms and in the way that you feel works best.

Before you begin

We've created a list of items for your purchase prior to starting the Fiber Fueled 4 Weeks. I recommend taking a day before getting started to go through your kitchen to see what you have and what you don't have. We don't want you to be halfway through the Fiber Fueled 4 Weeks and realize you need a piece of equipment that won't arrive for five days. And we want all the spices ready and handy. So we've created a Pre-FF4W checklist of items to get, including nonperishable foods and kitchen tools.

The philosophy behind the Fiber Fueled 4 Weeks

Alex is a registered dietitian, so not only does she know how to develop delicious recipes, but she's a nutrition expert who has completed the formal coursework, supervised internship, and national examination necessary to be qualified as an RD. Translation: She understands the science in great detail. You may have noticed that good science is really important to me. Yeah, I'm a nerd.

So what you're getting in the Fiber Fueled 4 Weeks goes so far beyond a bunch of plant-based recipes. There are layers of complexity that are built into the plan. Little tricks or strategies that Alex and I came up with to give you the optimal experience. But you don't need to worry, you just follow the plan, and in the process you get all of those benefits. It's our ninja way of delivering something powerful and cutting edge that's still straightforward and easy to follow.

In case you're interested in knowing what's going on behind the scenes, here's how it's going down: In Week 1, we're going to ease you into a plant-based diet with a one-week detox. These recipes were intentionally constructed with delicious plant foods that are also gentle on the gut. It gives you a chance to sweep out the junk of your old diet, ease into fiber and FODMAPs, and lay the foundation for a revitalized microbiome. We're not ignoring plant-based diversity, we're just moving slowly. Think of this as mild exercise. A brisk walk. A casual bike ride.

After that first week, it's time to start training our gut. We'll start with moderate exercise and ramp up over the course of the last three weeks. What I'm referring to here is the FODMAP content of our food. As we move through the Fiber Fueled 4 Weeks you'll be on a FODMAP progression. As I've said throughout the book, "Slow and low, that is the motto." We're also going to ramp up plant-based diversity. The addition of plant varieties translates into increased bacterial richness in our microbiome.

What to do with gluten?

Believe it or not, there isn't a ton of gluten in the Fiber Fueled 4 Weeks. The pancakes are gluten free, buckwheat doesn't actually contain wheat, and the bread is usually sourdough, which is pretty close to gluten free. But if you're strictly gluten free, make sure you keep that in mind going in so that you can make the appropriate substitutions as noted.

Why 28 days? Why not a quick 7- or 14-day detox?

I probably don't need to tell you this, but the length of the plan isn't some arbitrary period of time. Sure, it would've been easier to call it a detox and shorten it substantially, but you deserve better. A detox is a bridge to nowhere, and before long you return to your old habits and nothing's changed. Same for fad diets. This isn't a twenty-eight day plan that you do as an isolated event. This is a new beginning for you. We're laying the foundation of a revitalized microbiome and after the twenty-eight days you will be on the path to continuing what you started by living *Fiber Fueled*.

Research shows that it takes twenty-eight days for the microbiome to adapt to dietary fiber, get the digestive enzymes necessary for fiber processing, and increase SCFA production. The major changes occur within twenty-eight days, and after that things stay fairly stable. We also know that after antibiotics it takes about four weeks for the microbiota to approximate its pretreatment state. And in their study of TMAO, the Cleveland Clinic doctors found that it took about four weeks to ramp up TMAO production, and then four weeks for the microbiota to recover if you withdrew red meat from the diet. Four weeks keeps showing up as the magic amount of time.

This doesn't mean that your work is done after four weeks. Particularly if you have underlying dysbiosis, it may take longer to build up the strength of your microbiota and get to where you ultimately want to be. But science shows us that four weeks is around the time when the effort really starts to manifest in a powerful way. And *that* is why this is a Fiber Fueled 4 Weeks.

How to get the most out of the Fiber Fueled 4 Weeks

You are a unique individual! Literally no one in the world has a gut microbiome exactly like you, which means no one on the planet has the same taste buds or food sensitivities as you. You have your own starting point on this health journey, and you have your own goals for what you're trying to accomplish. Here are a few tips to maximize this journey for you:

Think of it as a culinary adventure

Over the next month, you'll be trying more than seventy new recipes for the first time. I'm sure there will be new flavors, new textures, and new ingredients. If you were traveling, you'd be taking day trips to Mexico, Italy, Greece, Turkey, India, Thailand, Korea, and Japan. Now that would be exhausting. So why not send your taste buds on this world tour while you are hanging in the comforts of your kitchen? And we still made time for American classics with a *Fiber Fueled* twist: Buffalo Chickpea Salad (page 301), No-Tuna Sunflower Salad (page 267) on sourdough, and New Orleans gumbo (see Gumbo, page 303).

Without a doubt, we love these recipes and can't wait to share them with you. I think you're going to love them, too! We want to offer you many different tastes so that you can discover where your plant passion lies. It's a jump start to the ultimate goal—an FF365 lifestyle. If you worry that you're not going to love these foods, don't worry. We've built enough variety into this plan to help you find something that you love. And the other thing is that your taste buds are definitely going to change. It happened for me, and it will happen for you, too.

I want you to keep a journal to track your journey during the FF4W. How did you feel about each recipe? Make notes and give each recipe a score from 0 to 10. Zero means it's just not for you, end of story. And if you give it a 10, that means you're salivating at the thought and jumping for joy when it's on the menu.

When the Fiber Fueled 4 Weeks is over, I want you to go back and pick out your three highest-rated breakfast dishes, five highest-rated lunches, and five highest-rated dinners. After our taste buds are done with their world tour during the four weeks, we ultimately want to settle in to real life and to have our "go-to" recipes that we use throughout the week. Not necessarily *every* week—you can use them however you feel is best. But the reality is that most of us have a rotation of core recipes, and during the Fiber Fueled 4 Weeks you're going to zero in on the dishes you like best.

You're Sherlock Holmes, food sensitivity sleuth

In Chapter 5 we talked about identifying the strengths and weaknesses in your gut, and using that information to train your gut by slowly introducing foods. In the FF4W plan, we're going to put that idea into action. Through our FODMAP progression we systematically introduce our healthiest and most challenging foods in a way that affords your gut an opportunity to start adapting to them. As you're going through this process, I'd like you to keep track of meals that cause GI distress—gas, bloating, discomfort, and change in bowel habits. Mark the meals in your journal that cause trouble so we can keep track.

I've offered a FODMAP note after recipes to help with this process. The note will explain what ingredients in a recipe have moderate or high FODMAP content, and it will offer guidance for substitutions. This will help you identify particular FODMAP categories you are most sensitive to (fructose, fructans, galactans, polyols, or mannitols). At the end of the FF4W you can look back in your journal to see what FODMAP categories were causing you the most trouble. This is empowering information since it will reveal where your food sensitivity lies. Over the course of time, you may eventually move past the low FODMAP option, which is proof that you're strengthening your gut.

If you email me at fodmap@theplantfedgut.com, I will send you a list of foods within each FODMAP category so that you can focus on the specific foods that contain a large amount of the FODMAP you are sensitive to and learn to moderate your portion size while you are training your gut.

The Fiber Fueled 4 Weeks is a great way to begin the process of identifying where your food sensitivity lies, but some of you with more advanced dysbiosis may require individualized assistance from a qualified health professional. The formal low FODMAP diet, including elimination and reintroduction, takes much longer than twenty-eight days. So if you're struggling even after doing the FF4W, I'd encourage you to meet with a registered dietitian and go through that process to work on the issue.

Your custom experience

The beauty of the Fiber Fueled 4 Weeks is that we're all sharing this collective journey, yet we have our own individualized experience. It has to be that way! We need a plan that's adapted to your bioindividuality. With that in mind, the plan is meant to be flexible. We *expect* you to bend the rules!

Each week you'll have recipes for drinks, snacks, and dessert. These are totally optional, meaning that you're under no obligation to make them but it's nice to have options for those things if you're in the mood. Of course, you can keep it super simple if you prefer and just snag a piece of fruit, some berries, or some nuts.

We give you a Quick Fix recipe for breakfast, lunch, and dinner each week. If at any point you're not able to cook, just sub in one of these recipes so you can keep rolling. Similarly, feel free to adapt recipes as you feel fit. Finally, try not to jump ahead in the schedule but feel free to bring back something that you've already tried.

The *Fiber Fueled* Challenge: Earn your plant points to reach the next level of health

Take your gut health to the next level by earning Plant Points at every meal. You'll find them attached to every recipe and proportional to plant diversity. This is a way to keep track of how you're doing. It's not a total number of plants for the week, but it's an easy way to keep track of total plant diversity—provided you don't eat the same eight plants at every meal!

The Plant Points will help you step your game up to supercharge your plant diversity. Over the course of the week, keep track of your

Plant Points in your journal. Add them up at the end of the week and punch them into the table below. It's totally okay if you start off on the low end of the spectrum. I was that guy not that long ago. By tracking your Plant Points, we're going to help you increase your plant diversity over time so you can graduate to the highest level. Tap into your inner plant-based rock star for inspiration to move up the following levels:

PLANT POINTS	WHAT LEVEL OF PLANT-BASED ROCK STAR ARE YOU?
Less than 150	**ROCK ROOKIE** You're just getting started and haven't felt the benefits yet, but I'm excited for you as you embark on this journey and start to feel the difference.
150–174	**ROCK ARTIST** You're starting to notice some changes. Your energy levels are higher, you're sleeping better, you don't feel hungover after meals. You may be working through some adjustments, but there are signs of progress.
175–199	**ROCK STAR** It's happening! Changes in the gut are under way and you are thriving on plant-based diversity with healthy bowel movements and better digestion.
200–224	**ROCK LEGEND** You are incredible! Pushing yourself to this level of plant-based diversity rewards you with a gut that feels amazing and is doing its job throughout the body to keep you well.
More than 225!	**ROCK GOD** You are a *Fiber Fueled* God of Rock with a microbiome that is wildly diversified and working like a well-oiled machine to keep you happy and healthy.

And the challenge doesn't end after four weeks! Sure, during your average week you don't need to keep track of Plant Points because with your "health mindset" you're maximizing plant-based diversity anyway. But every once in a while you may get an itch to have some fun and challenge yourself. When that happens, keep track of your points so you can compare it to prior scores and see how you do. Or even create a challenge on social media. Invite your friends or make some new friends! Let's get our *Fiber Fueled* community together for an online party. Tag me so I can be there cheering with you.

Calculate your own Plant Points

In case you're wondering, Plant Points are calculated by the number of plant foods included in the recipe. Every unique plant counts for one Plant Point. Pretty simple, right? Fresh herbs count, too, but dried herbs and spices don't. I still love them, though, and totally encourage you to liberally apply spices and enjoy the health benefits that ensue!

Integrating the Fiber Fueled 4 Weeks with the FF365 Lifestyle

As we get started on the Fiber Fueled 4 Weeks, make sure to keep in mind that this is more than a meal plan. We're building a lifestyle, galvanizing healthy habits, and using our "health mindset." So make sure to revisit the lifestyle elements discussed in Chapter 9 and start to incorporate those healthy habits into your routine. Multiple small changes can yield huge results. Our goal is to establish a baseline routine that leads to effortless fitness.

The last word

Before you take that first step into the Fiber Fueled 4 Weeks and what will be the rest of your life, I want you to know that I wholeheartedly believe in the power of the human spirit to persevere and overcome challenges. Nothing can stop the person with the fire inside them and the right attitude. So wherever you are coming from, if your mission is to heal your gut and recapture your health, I know you're going to do it and I'm so excited that the journey starts today and that this book will be a part of it for you.

PRE-FF4W CHECKLIST

To help things go smoothly, here is our list of appliances that you'll use throughout the weeks along with shelf-stable ingredients that might be hard to find, depending on your location, and therefore need to be ordered ahead of time.

- ☐ Slow cooker (see Notes)
- ☐ Blender
- ☐ Medium saucepan
- ☐ Small saucepan
- ☐ Rimmed baking sheet
- ☐ Food processor (see Notes)
- ☐ Muffin tin
- ☐ Large skillet
- ☐ Glass meal-prep containers
- ☐ Mix of glass storage containers, for leftovers
- ☐ Prep bowls, mix of sizes

Foods
- ☐ Dried shiitake mushrooms
- ☐ 2-ounce package kombu sheets
- ☐ Matcha powder (organic ceremonial grade)
- ☐ Nutritional yeast
- ☐ Gluten-free flour (Bob's Red Mill 1:1 and King Arthur Flour All-Purpose Gluten-Free Flour Mix are Week 1–approved)
- ☐ Garlic-infused olive oil (see page 246)

- ☐ Mushroom powder (see Mushroom Hot Cocoa on page 312 for more)
- ☐ Wakame seaweed

Herbs & Spices
- ☐ Ground ginger
- ☐ Ground cinnamon
- ☐ Ground nutmeg
- ☐ Salt (see Notes)
- ☐ Freshly ground black pepper
- ☐ Dried oregano
- ☐ Dried basil
- ☐ Dried parsley
- ☐ Crushed red pepper flakes, optional
- ☐ Ground turmeric
- ☐ Chili powder
- ☐ Smoked paprika
- ☐ Yellow curry powder
- ☐ Garam masala
- ☐ Ground cumin
- ☐ Vanilla extract
- ☐ Ground coriander
- ☐ Ground cayenne, optional
- ☐ Dried thyme
- ☐ Dried mustard
- ☐ Dried cardamom
- ☐ Garlic powder

Notes
- Slow cooker is only used in the recipe for Biome Broth (page 249), with an option for stove-top.
- If you don't own a food processor but have a good blender, then

you can use that in the recipes that call for a food processor, though you will likely have to remove the top, scrape down the sides, and blend a few times to get the same results.

- Since a plant-based diet can be low in iodine, we recommend using iodized salt to ensure you are getting a source of this vital nutrient. But if you're fermenting, make sure to use non-iodized salt.

Sunday Prep

Each week will begin with a meal-prep day to help cut down on cooking time later in the week. Spending a few hours at the start of the week will ensure that you're able to follow through with the twenty-eight-day meal plan, even when things get busy.

At the start of each week, you'll see a prep section highlighting the recommended and optional cooking steps. We've created this plan with efficiency in mind; that's why you'll see certain breakfasts, snacks, and desserts repeated throughout the plan. These are all items that are either simple to put together or can last for weeks at a time.

Drinks, Snacks, and Dessert

Being *Fiber Fueled* isn't about living in deprivation. It's about enjoying delicious food in abundance and *still* getting the results you want. With that in mind, every week we'll be offering a drink, two snacks, and two desserts to round out your culinary experience. You can sprinkle them into your routine as often as you desire. Keep in mind that if you love the Coconut Oat Balls (page 250) from Week 1, for example, you shouldn't hesitate to bring it back again in Week 3. As long as you don't jump ahead, you are totally free to reuse the recipes that you enjoy. Likewise, if you like having the same snack or dessert most days, that's fine, too!

Quick-Fix Recipes

Life can get the best of us sometimes. Some days you come home and just want to throw on your sweatpants and enjoy an easy peasy dinner that requires next to no effort. I totally get it! That's why we have Quick-Fix recommendations for each week. If you ever decide that you need something simple, you can opt for a Quick-Fix in place of the planned meal.

Week 1

Okay, folks, after all that reading and preparation, we are officially under way. You're going to be pushing yourself—trying new foods, new flavors, new cooking techniques. Embrace the challenge and share your experience online under the hashtag #fiberfueled4weeks. I'll be keeping an eye out for you and can't wait to cheer you on!

Remember, feel free to make adjustments as necessary to fit your tastes or your particular lifestyle. Don't forget to keep track of which recipes are your favorites, which you can do without, and if any meals make you sensitive.

WEEK 1 SHOPPING LIST
Produce
- ☐ 1 medium piece fresh ginger
- ☐ 7 large lemons
- ☐ 6 large red bell peppers
- ☐ 1 ounce dried shiitake mushrooms
- ☐ 1 pound carrots
- ☐ 1 pound celery hearts
- ☐ 1 pint cherry tomatoes
- ☐ One 5-ounce bag spinach leaves
- ☐ 3 kiwis
- ☐ 1 pound strawberries

- ☐ 2 bananas
- ☐ One 10-ounce package leafy salad greens
- ☐ 2 beets
- ☐ One 100-gram container broccoli sprouts
- ☐ 1 bunch fresh parsley
- ☐ 1 bunch fresh basil
- ☐ 1 large avocado
- ☐ 1 large eggplant
- ☐ 2 zucchini
- ☐ 7 Roma tomatoes
- ☐ 1 small fennel bulb
- ☐ 1 large pineapple
- ☐ 1 small bunch fresh chives
- ☐ 1 bunch kale (lacinato or curly)
- ☐ 1 jalapeño
- ☐ 1 bunch fresh cilantro
- ☐ 1 lime
- ☐ 1 pint blueberries
- ☐ 3 large sweet potatoes
- ☐ 2 parsnips
- ☐ 6 large radishes
- ☐ 2 bunches scallions
- ☐ 1 head romaine lettuce
- ☐ One 5-ounce container arugula
- ☐ 1 red chile pepper
- ☐ 1 head broccoli
- ☐ 2 heads bok choy
- ☐ 1 pound oyster mushrooms
- ☐ 2 large oranges
- ☐ 2 large salad tomatoes

Cupboard

☐ One 28-ounce jar peanut butter

☐ One 16-ounce container white miso paste

☐ One 16-ounce jar organic sunflower oil

☐ One 8-ounce container unsweetened cocoa powder

☐ One 28-ounce jar almond butter

☐ One 8-ounce bag unsweetened coconut flakes

☐ One 64-ounce container almond milk

☐ One 16-ounce bag chia seeds

☐ One 16-ounce bag hemp seeds

☐ One 16-ounce bag ground flaxseed

☐ Two 15-ounce cans chickpeas

☐ One 5-ounce jar sunflower kernels

☐ One 15-ounce jar tahini

☐ One 15-ounce can brown lentils

☐ One 24-ounce bag yellow cornmeal

☐ One 8-ounce bag unsweetened coconut flakes

☐ One 8-ounce bag dates

☐ One 4-ounce box wild rice

☐ One 30-ounce loaf sourdough bread

☐ One 8-ounce package tempeh

☐ One 16-ounce bag whole almonds

☐ Taco-size (small) corn tortillas (4)

☐ 1 pound firm tofu, packed in water

☐ One 8-ounce package rice noodles

☐ One 18-ounce container rolled oats

☐ One 3-ounce bag pepitas

☐ One 2.24-ounce can sliced black olives

☐ One 8-ounce package gluten-free pasta of choice

☐ One 8-ounce package quinoa

- ☐ One 15-ounce can coconut milk
- ☐ One 8-ounce package brown rice
- ☐ One 32-ounce container vegetable broth
- ☐ One 3-ounce can bamboo shoots
- ☐ One 20-ounce package arborio rice
- ☐ One 10-ounce bag chopped walnuts

Pantry Staples (If you don't have these on hand, grab them ahead of time)

- ☐ 100% maple syrup
- ☐ Balsamic vinegar
- ☐ Olive oil
- ☐ Ground cumin
- ☐ Sea salt
- ☐ Ground black pepper
- ☐ Crushed red pepper flakes
- ☐ Dried kombu
- ☐ Turmeric
- ☐ Tamari
- ☐ Nutritional yeast
- ☐ Vanilla extract
- ☐ Red wine vinegar
- ☐ Rice wine vinegar
- ☐ Pickling spice (or mustard seeds, cloves, and whole peppercorns)
- ☐ Apple cider vinegar
- ☐ Dried oregano
- ☐ Dried basil
- ☐ Chili powder
- ☐ Smoked paprika
- ☐ Cayenne pepper
- ☐ Italian scasoning
- ☐ Toasted sesame oil

☐ Cornstarch or arrowroot powder

☐ Ground ginger

☐ Ground cinnamon

☐ Ground nutmeg

☐ Dried cranberries, optional

☐ Yellow curry powder

☐ Garam masala powder

☐ Baking powder

☐ Baking soda

Week 1—Meal Prep

Week 1 Recommended Prep
Supercharged Roasted Roots (page 231)
Biome Broth (page 249)
Roasted Italian Medley (page 241)
Oil-Free Orange Dressing (page 230)
Muhammara Dip (page 248)
Crispy Oat Granola (page 228)
Coconut Oat Balls (page 250)
Zesty Lemon Chia Pudding (page 251)

Week 1 Optional Prep
Creamy Cilantro Sauce (page 237)
Berry Good Sweet Potato Toast (page 226)
Tempeh Taco Filling (page 236)

Week 1—Drinks, Snacks, and Dessert
Remember, these recipes are to be enjoyed whenever the moment feels right.
Drink Recipe: Lemon-Ginger Tea (page 247)
Snack Recipe #1: Muhammara Dip (page 248) with carrots and cu-
    cumbers

Snack Recipe #2: Miso Biome Sipper (page 249)
Dessert Recipe #1: Coconut Oat Balls (page 250)
Dessert Recipe #2: Zesty Lemon Chia Pudding (page 251)

Week 1—Quick-Fix Menu

When the going gets tough, no worries. Just opt for one of these recipes for super simple meals and snacks.

Friendly reminder: Berries can always be substituted for the dessert option if you prefer. To keep the berries low FODMAP this week, we recommend no more than ¼ cup blueberries or 10 strawberries at a time. More than that or other types of berries are considered high FODMAP for Week 1. More than 10 almonds is considered high FODMAP for Week 1.

Quick-Fix Breakfast: Superfood Smoothie (page 225)
Quick-Fix Lunch: Muhammara Sandwich (page 233)
Quick-Fix Dinner: Wild Biome Super Soup (page 232)
Quick-Fix Snack: 10 almonds
Quick-Fix Dessert: ¼ cup blueberries or 10 strawberries*

DAY 1 (USUALLY SUNDAY)

Friendly reminder: You can always substitute fruit for the snack or add extra fruit to your day.

Meal	Recipe	Page	Plant Points
Breakfast	Super Seedy Breakfast Porridge with Lemon-Ginger Tea	Porridge: 223 Lemon-Ginger Tea: 247	8

Lunch	The Daily Salad + Supercharged Roasted Roots + Oil-Free Orange Dressing	The Daily Salad: 229 Roasted Roots: 231	12
Dinner	Plant-Powered Polenta Ragu	235	8

DAY 2

Meal	Recipe	Page	Plant Points
Breakfast	Creamy Coconut Pudding with Pineapple	224	4
Lunch	Wild Biome Super Soup	Biome Broth: 249 Wild Biome Super Soup: 232	7+
Dinner	Tempeh Tacos	236	5+

DAY 3

Meal	Recipe	Page	Plant Points
Breakfast	Superfood Smoothie with Berry Good Sweet Potato Toast	Smoothie: 225 Toast: 226	9+
Lunch	Muhammara Sandwich	233	7
Dinner	Nourishing Tomato Noodle Soup with salad of leftover Supercharged Roasted Roots, lettuce, and Oil-Free Orange Dressing	Tomato soup: 238 Roasted roots: 231 Oil-Free Orange Dressing: 230	5–8

DAY 4

Meal	Recipe	Page	Plant Points
Breakfast	Super Seedy Breakfast Porridge	223	6
Lunch	Tempeh Taco Salad	236	5+
Dinner	Pesto Pasta with Roasted Italian Medley	Pesto pasta: 239 Italian veggies: 241	11

DAY 5

Meal	Recipe	Page	Plant Points
Breakfast	Berry Good Sweet Potato Toast	226	3–5
Lunch	The Daily Salad + Oil-Free Orange Dressing + sourdough toast and muhammara spread	229	13–18
Dinner	Back-Pocket Stir-Fry	242	7

DAY 6

Meal	Recipe	Page	Plant Points
Breakfast	Superfood Smoothie Bowl with Nut Butter Drizzle and Crispy Oat Granola	225	12
Lunch	Leftover Pesto Pasta with Down 'n' Dirty Kale Salad	Pesto pasta: 239 Kale salad: 233	11–13
Dinner	Curry Tofu Bok Choy	243	7–11

DAY 7

Meal	Recipe	Page	Plant Points
Breakfast	Gluten-Free Pancakes	262	2+
Lunch	Leftover Back-Pocket Stir-Fry	242	7
Dinner	Mushroom Risotto	245	5

BREAKFAST

Super Seedy Breakfast Porridge

This super seedy breakfast porridge is packed with ALA-rich hemp and chia seeds. While the ingredient list looks long, it's mostly spices and flavorings. If you have pumpkin pie spice on hand, you can use that instead of the ginger, cinnamon, and nutmeg.

For those who prefer a sweeter porridge, add maple syrup as desired. We like this best with fresh berries and a drizzle of almond butter on top.

Makes 2 servings
⅔ cup rolled oats
½ cup unsweetened almond milk
2 tablespoons raw pepitas, roughly chopped
Pinch ground ginger
Pinch ground cinnamon
Pinch ground nutmeg
2 tablespoons hemp seeds
1 tablespoon almond butter, plus more for serving
2 teaspoons chia seeds
½ teaspoon vanilla extract
100% maple syrup (optional)
Berries, for serving

Bring the oats and ⅔ cup water to a boil in a medium saucepan over medium-high heat. Reduce the heat to low and stir in the almond milk, pepitas, ginger, cinnamon, and nutmeg. Cook, stirring occasionally, for about 5 minutes, until the oats are tender.

Remove from the heat and stir in the hemp seeds, almond butter, chia seeds, and vanilla. Taste, adding maple syrup as desired for a sweeter porridge.

Serve with berries and additional almond butter drizzle, if desired.

6 PLANT POINTS

Creamy Coconut Pudding with Pineapple

We love the tropical pairing of pineapple and coconut, though other Week 1–friendly topping options include 30 raspberries or a heaping ¼ cup of blueberries.

Serves 2

2 cups unsweetened almond milk

¼ cup chia seeds

2 tablespoons ground flaxseed

1 tablespoon 100% maple syrup (optional)

1 teaspoon vanilla extract

2 tablespoons shredded, unsweetened coconut

2 cups sliced pineapple

1 date, chopped

Place the almond milk, chia seeds, flax meal, maple syrup, if using, and vanilla in a large mason jar with a lid and shake vigorously to combine. Place in the fridge for 20 minutes, then remove and shake again. Place back in the fridge for at least 30 minutes or up to overnight.

When ready to serve, divide into two bowls, stir in the coconut, and top with pineapple and chopped date.

Low FODMAP Option:

Decrease the total quantity of pineapple to 1 cup.

Dates are a high FODMAP food, so in Week 1, limit your serving size to ⅓ chopped date per serving. In Week 2, increase your serving size to ½ date. After Week 3, if dates are not a trigger food, you can consume a full date.

Packing Tip:
Make this in your favorite glass container with a lid in the evening, add the toppings in the morning, and pack this to take with you on busy mornings!

4 PLANT POINTS

Superfood Smoothie, with Bowl Option

We call this a "superfood" smoothie for good reason—it's packed with all of the good stuff: ALA-rich hemp seeds, spinach, broccoli sprouts, berries, and satisfying peanut butter. If you prefer your smoothie on the sweeter side, you may need a touch of maple syrup for Weeks 1 and 2. From there, feel free to add in more berries or kiwi and omit the sweetener altogether.

Serves 1
1 cup almond milk
2 tablespoons hemp seeds
½ cup spinach leaves
Small handful broccoli sprouts
1 kiwi, skin removed
5 medium strawberries
2 tablespoons peanut butter
½ frozen banana
1 to 2 teaspoons 100% maple syrup (optional)

Place all ingredients in a blender and puree until very smooth and creamy. Depending on the power of your blender, you may need to add more liquid.

To make a smoothie bowl, reduce the liquid by half (use ½ cup almond milk), then blend as directed. Divide the contents into two bowls and drizzle with peanut butter and top with more berries, if desired. Garnish with more fresh fruit, seeds, nut butter, and Crispy Oat Granola (page 228).

Packing Tip:

Place the smoothie or bowl in a mason jar with a lid or leak-proof container with a lid. For the bowl, pack toppings in a separate leak-proof container, then combine once ready to eat.

Low FODMAP Option:

Unripe bananas are lower in FODMAPs than ripe bananas. Half a ripe banana or 1 medium unripe banana are both low FODMAP. Use ½ banana if you are sensitive to fructose.

6 PLANT POINTS

Berry Good Sweet Potato Toast

While we are big fans of sourdough, this sweet potato version is a nice way to mix up French toast. We're serving it with almond butter and blueberries, but the topping choices are endless after Week 1. This recipe also includes make-ahead prep for parbaking the sweet potatoes ahead of time, then popping them into a toaster when ready to eat.

You'll need a sharp knife to cut the potatoes into slabs, or you can use a mandoline for more uniform slices.

Makes 10 or 11 slices
1 large sweet potato, washed and dried
2 tablespoons almond butter
20 blueberries

Preheat the oven to 350°F. Place a wire rack on a large rimmed baking sheet and set aside.

Trim both ends from the sweet potato using a knife, then slice the potato lengthwise into ¼-inch-thick slabs using a knife or mandoline.

Place the slabs onto the wire rack (or directly onto the baking sheet) in a single layer and place in the middle of the oven. Cook for 15 to 20 minutes, until the potatoes are tender but not fully cooked, checking every 5 minutes to make sure they don't burn. Thinner potatoes will need less cooking time and thicker potatoes will need more. If you aren't using a wire rack, flip the potatoes halfway through.

Remove from the oven and allow to cool completely on the wire rack, then transfer to an airtight container and store in the fridge for up to 4 days.

When ready to serve, place the sweet potato slices (about 2 slices is a good serving size) in a toaster or toaster oven on the medium setting and toast until hot and the edges are crispy (the cook time required will depend on your toaster). Serve with almond butter and blueberries.

Low FODMAP Option:

For the first week, limit your sweet potato portion size to ½ cup (4 ounces). This will keep the sweet potato in a low FODMAP portion size.

Supercharge It!

Add a dash of cinnamon, a sprinkle of unsweetened coconut flakes, or even a few hemp seeds on top of this toast for more Plant Points and nutrients.

3 PLANT POINTS

Crispy Oat Granola

This granola is the perfect topper for smoothies and smoothie bowls. We also love noshing on this crispy, subtly sweet granola with a touch of plant-based milk or on its own. While the cranberries are an optional add-in, we are obsessed with their tart, sweet flavor and chewy texture!

Makes 4¼ cups
2 cups rolled oats
1 cup unsweetened, shredded coconut
1 cup chopped walnuts
2 tablespoons chia seeds
2 tablespoons hemp seeds
2 tablespoons ground flaxseed
1 teaspoon ground cinnamon
¾ teaspoon salt
2 tablespoons organic sunflower oil
¼ cup 100% maple syrup
1 teaspoon vanilla extract
½ cup dried cranberries (optional)

Preheat the oven to 250°F. Line a rimmed baking sheet with parchment.

In a large bowl, combine the oats, coconut, walnuts, chia seeds, hemp seeds, flaxseed, cinnamon, and salt.

In a small saucepan over medium heat, whisk the sunflower oil into the maple syrup. Bring to a simmer, then remove from the heat and add the vanilla.

Add the syrup mixture to the oat ingredients and mix thoroughly. Spread the granola in a single layer on the prepared baking sheet. Bake for 90 minutes, stirring every 15 minutes, until golden brown.

Cool completely, then stir in the dried cranberries, if using. Transfer to an airtight container and store for several weeks in the fridge, or in the freezer for up to 3 months.

Make-Ahead Tips:

This dish makes quite a bit. We suggest making this at the start of Week 1 and enjoying it throughout the meal plan. Store in an airtight container to prevent it from drying out.

Low FODMAP Option:

1 tablespoon dried cranberries per serving is low FODMAP.

6 PLANT POINTS

LUNCH

The Daily Salad

We call this the daily salad because we believe in the power of eating raw vegetables every single day, and what better way than a *Fiber Fueled* salad? If you're looking for a filling, satisfying, and easy-to-throw-together option, this is it. We call for pickled beets in this recipe. They're low FODMAP even though plain beets are fairly high.

Serves 2

Salad

4 cups chopped leafy greens

½ cup Quick-Pickled Beets (recipe follows), or store-bought

½ cup cooked chickpeas

¼ cup sunflower seeds

Handful broccoli sprouts

1 medium carrot, shredded

10 cherry tomatoes, sliced

Oil-Free Orange Dressing

¼ cup freshly squeezed orange juice

2 tablespoons apple cider vinegar

2 tablespoons tahini

¼ teaspoon salt, plus more to taste

¼ teaspoon freshly ground black pepper, plus more to taste

Supercharged Roasted Roots (optional; recipe follows), for serving

Make the salad: In a large bowl, toss together the greens, pickled beets, chickpeas, sunflower seeds, sprouts, carrots, tomatoes, and any other Supercharge toppings, if using. Set aside.

Make the dressing: Whisk together the orange juice, vinegar, tahini, salt, and pepper in a small bowl or mason jar until smooth. Starting with 1 tablespoon at a time, whisk in water until your desired consistency is reached (the dressing should be pourable but not runny). Add salt and pepper, as desired. If using later, the dressing will keep in the fridge for up to 5 days.

When ready to serve, drizzle each salad with ¼ cup dressing, toss well, and add salt and pepper to taste.

Supercharge It!

Add 1 cup Supercharged Roasted Roots (page 231), chopped parsley, and cubed, baked tofu. After Week 2, you can top with ½ avocado.

9 PLANT POINTS

Quick-Pickled Beets

2 cups steamed, sliced beets

¼ cup plus 2 tablespoons red wine vinegar

1 tablespoon 100% maple syrup

1 tablespoon pickling spice (see Note)

Place the cooked beets, vinegar, maple syrup, and pickling spice in a small saucepan and bring to a boil over high heat. Reduce the heat to a simmer, cover, and let cook for 3 minutes. Remove from the heat and let sit for 30 minutes.

Refrigerate the beets for up to 1 week in the fridge.

Note: If you don't have pickling spice, you can use a pinch of mustard seeds, 2 or 3 whole cloves, and a pinch of whole peppercorns instead.

Supercharged Roasted Roots

This topping is designed to supercharge your meals wherever you want a little fiber boost. Add a handful to salads, Nourishing Buddha Bowls (page 295), or Tofu Scramble Bowls (page 286), or just enjoy them on their own.

This mix is perfect for Week 1, but the technique can be used on almost any vegetable out there, though cooking times may need to be adjusted.

Serves 4

2 cups cubed sweet potato

2 parsnips, chopped

6 large radishes, chopped

1 tablespoon olive oil, or garlic-infused olive oil (see page 246)

2 tablespoons vegetable broth

½ teaspoon salt

½ teaspoon freshly ground pepper

Preheat the oven to 425°F.

Toss the sweet potato, parsnips, radishes, olive oil, broth, salt, and pepper together in a large bowl until well combined. Place on a rimmed baking sheet in a single layer (you may need to use two, depending on size) and cover with foil.

Roast for 35 minutes, or until mostly soft. Remove from the oven, remove the foil, and stir. Return to the oven for 10 more minutes, or until the edges become lightly crisp.

3 PLANT POINTS

Wild Biome Super Soup

Wild rice and chickpeas make this hearty soup delicious and satisfying. While you can enjoy this soup any time of year, it's very comforting and perfect for a cold and rainy day.

Makes 2 servings
1 teaspoon olive oil
2 carrots, chopped
1 celery stalk, chopped
2 tablespoons fresh chives, chopped
¼ teaspoon salt, plus more to taste
⅛ teaspoon freshly ground black pepper, plus more to taste
2½ cups Biome Broth (page 249)
⅓ cup wild rice
½ cup chickpeas
1 cup kale, stems removed and roughly chopped

In a medium saucepan, heat the olive oil over medium-high heat. Add the carrots, celery, chives, salt, and pepper. Cook for 3 to 5 minutes, until the vegetables are crisp-tender.

Add in the broth, rice, and ½ cup water. Bring the mixture to a boil, then cover and reduce the heat to low. Simmer for about 40 minutes, until the rice has softened.

Mix in the chickpeas and kale and cook until the kale is just wilted, about 5 minutes. Add salt and pepper to taste.

Packing Tip:
Pack in a thermos to enjoy warm at work or place in a leak-proof container and warm right before serving. We like Bklyn Bento jars, which come with a bamboo spoon, or Lillie Home stainless-steel thermoses.

Supercharge It!
Serve this with a side of sourdough bread and the Muhammara Dip (page 248) you have made from the meal plan. Top with freshly chopped scallions.

7 PLANT POINTS

Muhammara Sandwich

To pack this sandwich for lunch, pack the toast, roasted Italian vegetables, spinach, and dip separately, then combine right before eating. We enjoy this as an open-faced sandwich.

Makes 1 sandwich
Leftover Muhammara Dip (page 248)
Leftover Roasted Italian Medley (page 241)
Sourdough bread
Fresh spinach leaves

Right before serving, toast the bread and warm the dip and vegetables. Spread the muhammara dip on both pieces of the bread, then layer with vegetables and spinach leaves. Eat as an open-faced sandwich, or assemble, slice, and enjoy.

7 PLANT POINTS

Down 'n' Dirty Kale Salad

This is one of our favorite ways to enjoy kale! The avocado–almond butter dressing is creamy and bursting with flavor. Simple to make, filled with flavor and texture, and brimming with plant-powered nutrients! We use this one as a side dish for multiple meals throughout the four-week plan.

Serves 2

1 heaping cup kale (dinosaur is best), tough stems removed and chopped

3 teaspoons low-sodium tamari

1 heaping cup spinach

2 tablespoons chives

¼ teaspoon salt

⅛ teaspoon freshly ground black pepper

¼ avocado, mashed

2 tablespoons almond butter

½ stalk celery, chopped

2 tablespoons walnuts, roughly chopped (optional)

¼ cup chopped scallions (green parts only) (optional)

In a medium bowl, drizzle the kale with 1 teaspoon tamari and massage with your hands to soften and break down the kale. Add the spinach, chives, salt, and pepper and toss together once more.

In a separate small bowl, mash the avocado with the almond butter and whisk in the remaining 2 teaspoons of tamari to thin.

Pour the avocado mixture over the kale and combine thoroughly with your hands or with tongs, massaging to coat every piece.

Add the celery, walnuts, and scallions and serve.

FODMAP Alternative Suggestions:

If you can tolerate a higher portion than ½ cup, increase your serving of kale, as this recipe makes a lot of dressing!

Make-Ahead Tips:

This salad tastes good a day after making, but not much longer. If you plan on making a portion to enjoy now and enjoying the second portion later, only dress half the greens with half of the dressing and toppings. Store the

remaining kale, spinach, dressing, chopped celery, walnuts, and scallions separately until ready to enjoy.

5 PLANT POINTS

DINNER

Plant-Powered Polenta Ragu

Creamy polenta is stick-to-your-ribs comfort food, especially when combined with our quick ragu of Italian vegetables and lentils. After Week 1, try this ragu with Pepita Parmesan (page 301), a nutty parm that's delicious on everything from pasta to polenta to popcorn.

Serves 2

Quick Ragu

2 teaspoons olive oil, garlic-infused olive oil (see page 246), or vegetable broth

1 cup chopped tomatoes

Salt and freshly ground black pepper

1 cup canned lentils

2 cups Roasted Italian Medley (page 241)

½ teaspoon dried oregano, plus more to taste

½ teaspoon dried basil, plus more to taste

Crushed red pepper flakes (optional)

Polenta

1½ cups plain almond milk

½ cup cornmeal

½ teaspoon salt

Freshly ground black pepper

Chopped parsley, for serving

Chopped fresh basil, for serving

Make the ragu: Heat a medium saucepan over medium heat and add the olive oil. Add in the tomatoes and a pinch of salt and black pepper. Cook, stirring often, for about 10 minutes, until the tomatoes have broken down. Add the lentils, Roasted Italian Medley, oregano, basil, and red pepper flakes, if using. Cook, stirring occasionally, for 10 minutes, or until thickened. Taste as you go and add more salt, pepper, and dried herbs as desired.

Make the polenta: Whisk together ½ cup water and the almond milk in a medium saucepan over medium heat. When bubbles start to surface, whisk in the cornmeal and salt. Reduce the heat to a simmer and cook for 10 to 15 minutes, until thickened. Taste as you go and add more salt and pepper to taste.

To serve, divide the polenta into two bowls and top with the ragu. Garnish with fresh chopped parsley and basil.

8 PLANT POINTS

Tempeh Tacos and Taco Salad

The tempeh taco filling and creamy cilantro sauce are designed to do double-duty in both the tacos and taco salad. Save time by making the entire batch, then portioning half to save for later in the week.

Serves 4
Tempeh Taco Filling
1 tablespoon olive oil
8 ounces tempeh, finely chopped
1 tablespoon chili powder
2 teaspoons smoked paprika
½ teaspoon salt
¼ teaspoon ground cayenne pepper
1 cup canned lentils, drained

Creamy Cilantro Sauce

1 jalapeño, roughly chopped

½ bunch cilantro

¼ cup slivered almonds

Zest and juice of 1 lime

1 teaspoon salt

For Tacos

4 corn tortillas

Shredded lettuce, black olives, chopped tomatoes, scallions, and cilantro, for serving

For Salad

4 cups shredded lettuce

½ cup chopped tomatoes

⅓ cup sliced black olives

2 sliced scallions (green parts only)

⅓ cup chopped cilantro

Make the taco filling: Heat the oil in a large skillet over medium heat. Add the tempeh. Use a wooden spoon to break it into small pieces, then add in the chili powder, smoked paprika, salt, and cayenne pepper. Cook for about 10 minutes, until the tempeh is softened, adding a splash of broth or water if the tempeh sticks to the pan or gets too dry. Add the lentils and stir to combine and warm through.

Make the creamy cilantro sauce: Place the jalapeño, cilantro, almonds, lime zest, lime juice, ½ cup water, and the salt into a blender and puree until creamy and smooth. The consistency should be similar to a thick salad dressing. Add more water, 1 tablespoon at a time, if the dressing is too thick.

Assemble the tacos: Right before serving, warm the tortillas. Add half of the tempeh filling to the corn tortillas and top with shredded lettuce, tomatoes, olives, scallions, cilantro, and dressing.

Reserve the remaining half of the filling for taco salad later in the week.

Assemble the taco salad: Toss together the lettuce, tomatoes, olives, scallions, and cilantro and divide into two bowls. Top with the remaining tempeh taco filling and drizzle with the cilantro dressing.

Make-Ahead Tip:

Prep the tempeh taco filling and creamy cilantro sauce ahead of time, up to 3 days before serving. Portion half of the tempeh taco filling and creamy cilantro dressing to use later in the week for Tempeh Taco Salad.

Low FODMAP Option:

Chili powder may contain garlic, so make sure to read the ingredient list and pay attention to how you feel after this meal.

5+ PLANT POINTS

Nourishing Tomato Noodle Soup

Tomato noodle soup for this soul. This low FODMAP soup is comforting, nourishing, and just plain delicious.

Serves 2

3 cups Biome Broth (page 249), plus more as needed

1 scallion (green part only), sliced

2 teaspoons freshly grated ginger

1 Roma tomato, finely diced

1 tablespoon tamari

6 ounces firm tofu, drained, lightly pressed (see Note), and finely cubed

½ teaspoon ground turmeric

5 ounces rice noodles

2 teaspoons miso paste

1 teaspoon toasted sesame oil (optional)

Supercharged Roasted Roots (optional; page 231), for serving

Heat 2 tablespoons of the broth in a medium saucepan over medium heat. Add in the scallion greens, ginger, tomato, and tamari and cook for about 10 minutes, until the tomato is well broken down. Add a splash or two of broth as needed.

Add the tofu and cook 1 to 2 more minutes, stirring occasionally to prevent sticking. Add the turmeric and the remaining broth, then bring to a low boil. Let simmer for 10 minutes for the flavors to develop.

Reduce the heat to a simmer, then add in the rice noodles. Cook for another 2 or 3 minutes, until the noodles are tender and cooked through.

Turn off the heat and stir in the miso. Drizzle with sesame oil, if using, and top with the roasted roots to serve, if desired.

Supercharge It!

Top with 1 slice toasted nori, cut into strips, sesame seeds, and sliced scallion greens.

5 PLANT POINTS

Note: To press tofu, slice into slabs, then wrap in clean kitchen towels or paper towels. Place on a rimmed baking sheet, then cover with a heavy object, such as food cans or a skillet. Let sit for 10 minutes, until much of the water is removed.

Pesto Pasta

This hearty pasta dinner comes together quickly, using the leftover Roasted Italian Medley (page 241) from earlier in the week.

Serves 4

Arugula-Walnut Pesto

3 cups packed arugula

½ cup lightly toasted walnuts

2 tablespoons nutritional yeast

2 tablespoons freshly squeezed lemon juice

¼ cup vegetable broth or water

¼ teaspoon salt, plus more to taste

¼ teaspoon freshly ground black pepper, plus more to taste

1 tablespoon olive oil (optional)

8 ounces dried gluten-free pasta

2 cups Roasted Italian Medley (recipe follows)

Make the pesto: Place the arugula, walnuts, and nutritional yeast in the base of a food processor and blend until very finely chopped. With the motor running, add in the lemon juice, vegetable broth, salt, and pepper. Add more salt and pepper to taste. Drizzle in the olive oil, if using, and set aside.

Bring a large pot of salted water to a boil. Add the pasta and cook until just al dente according to package directions. Reserve ½ cup of pasta water and drain the pasta.

Place the pasta back into the pot along with the pesto. Toss, adding splashes of pasta water as needed to coat the pasta. Stir in the leftover Roasted Italian Medley and serve. If you prefer your pasta a little spicy, enjoy this with crushed red pepper flakes.

Low FODMAP Options:

Ancient Harvest and NOW Foods both have great quinoa pasta.

Chickpea pasta is also good, but has moderate FODMAP with over a
1-cup serving.

If tolerated after Week 3, add in 1 or 2 garlic cloves to the pesto.

If tolerated after Week 2, top with Pepita Parmesan (page 301).

6 PLANT POINTS

Roasted Italian Medley

This one-pan side dish is designed to make meal prep for Week 1 even easier. You'll use these vegetables over and over again in different ways: in the Plant-Powered Polenta Ragu (page 235), the Muhammara Sandwich (page 233), and the Pesto Pasta (239).

Makes 6 cups
1 large eggplant, cubed
2 medium zucchini, diced
1 red bell pepper, seeded and cubed
2 Roma tomatoes, diced
1 small fennel (1½ cups), fronds removed and diced
1 teaspoon dried Italian seasoning
¼ cup vegetable broth
2 to 3 teaspoons olive oil
½ teaspoon salt
½ teaspoon freshly ground black pepper
¼ teaspoon crushed red pepper flakes (optional)

Preheat the oven to 400°F.

In a large bowl, toss together the eggplant, zucchini, bell pepper, Roma tomatoes, fennel, Italian seasoning, vegetable broth, olive oil, salt, black pepper, and red pepper flakes, if using. Place in a single layer on a rimmed baking sheet (you may need two baking sheets, depending on the size), then place on the top rack of the oven.

Cook for 35 to 40 minutes, depending on the size of your vegetables, until the vegetables are very tender.

Keep in the fridge for up to 6 days. Enjoy any extras as is, on salads, or combined with cooked whole-grain pasta.

Low FODMAP Options:

Fennel has moderate mannitols and fructans. Less than ½ cup is considered low FODMAP.

5 PLANT POINTS

Back-Pocket Stir-Fry

Simplicity wins here. This stir-fry is made for Week 1 but simple enough to mix and match with other vegetables after the first week. Instead of a traditional protein source, we're serving this over quinoa, a pseudo-grain that packs in 8 grams of protein and 5 grams of fiber per cup. Enjoy leftovers for lunch later in the week.

Serves 4

⅓ cup tamari

¼ cup rice wine vinegar

2 tablespoons toasted sesame oil

2 teaspoons cornstarch or arrowroot

¼ cup Biome Broth (page 249) or water

2 tablespoons freshly grated ginger

1 red chile, seeded and minced (optional)

4 scallions (green parts only), sliced

2 cups broccoli florets only, chopped

4 carrots, sliced on the bias

1 red bell pepper, sliced

2 cups bok choy, sliced, leaves and stems separated

8 ounces oyster mushrooms, sliced

4 cups cooked quinoa, for serving

In a small bowl, whisk together the tamari, vinegar, sesame oil, and cornstarch until smooth. Set aside.

Heat the broth in a large skillet or wok over medium-high heat. Add the ginger, chili, if using, and sliced scallions. Cook, stirring often, until fragrant, about 1 minute.

Add the broccoli, carrots, bell pepper, and bok choy stems and cook, stirring often, for 5 to 7 minutes, until the vegetables are bright in color and slightly tender. Add in the bok choy leaves and oyster mushrooms and stir together for 30 seconds.

Add the tamari mixture to the wok. Cook, stirring often, until the sauce has thickened and the vegetables are cooked through.

Serve over cooked quinoa.

Low FODMAP Option:

After Week 2, add 1 or 2 minced garlic cloves to the tamari mixture.

7 PLANT POINTS

Curry Tofu Bok Choy

This simple dinner combines two of our favorite plant-powered foods: calcium- and iron-rich tofu and bok choy. Baby bok choy is more tender than the bigger bok choy, so if you prefer a milder vegetable, select that one instead.

Makes 2 servings

1¼ cups plus 2 tablespoons vegetable broth or Biome Broth (page 249), plus more as needed

½ cup canned coconut milk

1 tablespoon yellow curry powder

1 tablespoon garam masala powder

2 scallions (green parts only), thinly sliced

1 tablespoon freshly grated ginger

1 tablespoon tamari

3 cups bok choy, leaves and stems separated

3 ounces canned bamboo shoots (rinsed)

7 ounces firm tofu, pressed and cubed (see page 259)

1 teaspoon toasted sesame oil

1¼ cups cooked brown rice, for serving

In a medium bowl, whisk together 1¼ cups vegetable broth, the coconut milk, yellow curry powder, and garam masala until the spices are thoroughly mixed in. Set aside.

Heat the remaining 2 tablespoons broth in a large skillet or wok over medium-high heat until shimmering. Add the scallions, ginger, and tamari. Stir for about 1 minute, until the mixture is fragrant and the ginger is mostly broken down.

Add in the bok choy stems and bamboo shoots and sauté for about 5 minutes, until softened. If you need more liquid, add in a splash or two of the broth.

Toss the tofu with the sesame oil and set aside. Add to the wok and stir for 30 seconds to incorporate with the bok choy and bamboo shoots.

Reduce the heat to medium-low and add the coconut milk mixture and remaining bok choy leaves. Cover and reduce the heat to low. Let simmer for about 10 minutes, until the sauce is thickened and vegetables are tender and cooked through. Serve over cooked rice.

Make-Ahead Tips:

Chop the scallions and bok choy prior to cooking. Store in a sealed container in the fridge. This entire dish can be made ahead of time, cooled, and stored in a sealed container in the fridge, then reheated when you are ready to enjoy!

Low FODMAP Options:

Read the ingredient label and make sure your curry powder and garam masala do not contain garlic or onion.

Supercharge It!

Top with chopped cilantro, sesame seeds, and/or bean sprouts.

7 PLANT POINTS

Mushroom Risotto

Yes, risotto takes a little more time than other meals to make, but the constant stirring is like meditation to us. Put on a podcast (*Plant Proof* and *Party in My Plants* are my faves!) and enjoy standing over the stove, creating a warm bowl of delicious, creamy rice. Thirty minutes later you are rewarded with a rich, luxurious risotto dish without any cream, cheese, or butter. You're welcome!

Serves 4

4 cups Biome Broth (page 249) or FODMAP-friendly vegetable broth

2 tablespoons garlic-infused olive oil (see Note)

8 ounces oyster mushrooms, chopped

Salt

1¼ cups arborio or other short-grain rice

1 tablespoon freshly squeezed lemon juice

3 tablespoons nutritional yeast

Fresh parsley or fresh chives, chopped, for serving

In a small saucepot, heat the vegetable broth over medium heat. Once simmering, reduce the heat to low to keep warm.

While the broth is heating, heat a separate large saucepan over medium heat. Once hot, add in 1 tablespoon olive oil and heat until just shimmering, then add the mushrooms and a pinch of salt. Sauté for about 10 minutes, until tender and browned. Remove from the pan and set aside.

Heat the remaining 1 tablespoon of oil in the saucepan and add the rice. Cook, stirring often, for 1 minute until just lightly toasted. Using a ladle, add in the warmed vegetable broth, ½ cup at a time, stirring almost constantly, allowing the rice to absorb all of the liquid. Take care not to boil the mixture, as that will result in gummy risotto; the heat should be no higher than medium, with the mixture at a slight simmer.

Continue to add in the vegetable broth, ½ cup at a time, stirring to incorporate until the liquid is mostly absorbed before adding in more broth. The whole process should take about 20 minutes, until the rice is al dente.

Add the lemon juice, nutritional yeast, and reserved mushrooms, stirring to combine. Depending on your broth, you likely don't need any more salt, but season to taste as desired. Serve with chopped parsley or chives, as desired.

Note: When eating low FODMAP, garlic is avoided because it is high in fructans. Garlic-infused olive oil has the green light for a low FODMAP diet because the fructans are not lipid soluble so they will not leach into the oil. Just make sure to only consume the oil and don't eat the garlic. Fody Foods makes a great garlic-infused olive oil or you can make your own. Crush a few garlic cloves to break the skin—you'll need about 1 cup of olive oil for 5 to 6 garlic cloves. Gently heat the oil and garlic over low to medium heat for a few minutes, then allow the oil to cool. Remove the garlic, then store the oil in the fridge.

Low FODMAP Options:

For a store-bought, low FODMAP vegetable broth, try brands such as Fody Foods, Savory Choice, or Casa de Santé.

Oyster mushrooms are recommended in Week 1 as they are low

FODMAP. Substitute other mushrooms with caution in Week 1, as they contain mannitol and fructans.

After Week 2 and if okay with garlic and onions, sauté 1 cup chopped onion and 2 minced garlic cloves in the pan after you remove the mushrooms and before you add the rice.

5 PLANT POINTS

SNACKS, DESSERTS, AND DRINKS

Lemon-Ginger Tea

We like this lemon-ginger tea as an after-dinner drink. Ginger aids in digestion, and lemon contains just enough pucker to satisfy any dessert cravings. Feel free to drink it liberally, whenever you feel it suits you.

Serves 2

1 small ginger knob, sliced into four 1-inch chunks
Juice of 1 large lemon
100% maple syrup or stevia, as desired

In a medium saucepan, simmer 4 cups water and the ginger for 10 to 15 minutes, or longer, depending on how strong you like your tea.

Remove from the heat and stir in the lemon juice. Strain, removing the ginger, and divide the tea between 2 large mugs. Stir in the maple syrup and serve.

To serve cold: Pour the ginger-water mixture over 4 cups of ice and add the lemon juice and maple syrup, as desired.

2 PLANT POINTS

Muhammara Dip

Muhammara, made from roasted red peppers, walnuts, cumin, and red pepper flakes, is a hot pepper dip with Syrian roots. We love this smoky spread with vegetables and toasted sourdough, and in our Muhammara Sandwich (page 243).

Makes about 2½ cups dip
6 large red bell peppers
1 cup raw walnuts, chopped
2 tablespoons olive oil
¼ cup freshly squeezed lemon juice
¼ cup balsamic vinegar
1 teaspoon ground cumin
1 teaspoon sea salt, plus more to taste
½ teaspoon crushed red pepper flakes (or more, for a spicy dip)

Preheat the oven to 450°F.

Place the whole bell peppers directly onto a rimmed baking sheet and roast for 25 minutes, turning after 15 minutes, so that the bell peppers are lightly charred on each side.

Place the peppers in a large bowl and immediately cover with a kitchen towel to allow them to steam for at least 10 minutes. This will help the skin soften so it's easier to remove.

Once cool, remove the skin, core, and seeds. Roughly chop and set aside.

To the base of a food processor, add in the walnuts, olive oil, lemon juice, vinegar, cumin, salt, and red pepper flakes. Pulse 8 to 10 times to combine. Add in the roasted peppers and pulse a few more times to combine. You can make this into a creamy, hummus-like spread or a chunky nut spread. Taste and adjust as needed, adding more lemon for acidity, chili flakes for spice, balsamic vinegar for depth, and/or salt.

This will keep, covered, in the fridge for up to 4 days.

3 PLANT POINTS

Biome Broth

This broth tames inflammation, nourishes your gut, and packs some stellar antioxidants. We recommend making a batch every Sunday using a slow cooker for easy prep. As the weeks progress, feel free to add in more aromatics, like onion and garlic, for a more robust broth. Start with 1 chopped onion and 2 garlic cloves and adjust from there.

For a quick snack, warm up a cup (or two!) of this broth and stir in a tablespoon of miso paste until dissolved. Sip as is, or throw in cubed tofu, chopped scallions, and/or roasted mushrooms and steamed kale.

Makes about 8 cups
1 large piece dried kombu
1 cup chopped carrots
1 cup chopped celery
⅓ cup dried shiitake mushrooms or 1 teaspoon mushroom powder
1-inch piece fresh ginger, sliced
2 tablespoons nutritional yeast
2 tablespoons olive oil
3 tablespoons tamari
¼ teaspoon ground turmeric
Miso Biome Sipper
2 cups Biome Broth
2 teaspoons freshly grated ginger
2 teaspoons miso paste

Place the kombu, carrots, celery, mushrooms, ginger, nutritional yeast, olive oil, tamari, turmeric, and 8 cups water in a slow cooker and simmer on low for at least 6 hours. Alternatively, place in a large stockpot and simmer on low for at least 2 hours, stirring occasionally.

Let cool, then strain through a fine-mesh strainer. Divide into glass containers, placing some in the freezer for use later in the week and some in the fridge for immediate use. Make sure, if freezing in a glass container, to leave plenty of room for the liquid to expand. If not, the glass could break!

To make the miso biome sipper, warm the broth over medium heat, then remove from the heat and stir in the ginger and miso paste until dissolved, about 30 seconds. Divide into two mugs and sip.

Supercharge It!

Add ½ teaspoon mushroom powder to the biome sipper as you warm the broth. Top with sliced scallion greens.

6 PLANT POINTS

Coconut Oat Balls

Makes about 14 balls, depending on size

1 cup old-fashioned oats, plus more as needed

⅓ cup unsweetened coconut flakes

⅓ cup peanut butter, plus more as needed

2 tablespoons 100% maple syrup

2 tablespoons chia seeds

1 teaspoon vanilla extract

¼ teaspoon ground cinnamon

1 ounce finely chopped dark chocolate

Place the oats, coconut flakes, peanut butter, maple syrup, chia seeds, vanilla, and cinnamon in the base of a food processor and pulse 10 to 12 times, until just combined (you can also just mix these ingredients together in a large mixing bowl until thoroughly combined). If the mixture is too sticky to roll into balls, add some more oats. If it's too dry, add in more peanut butter.

Add the dark chocolate and pulse to just combine.

Pinch off a 1-tablespoon ball using either a spoon or small cookie scoop. Roll into a ball, then continue with the rest of the mixture. Store in an airtight container for 1 week or in the freezer for up to 3 months.

FODMAP notes:

While all of the ingredients here are lower FODMAP, stick to 2 balls per serving.

4 PLANT POINTS

Zesty Lemon Chia Pudding

This lemon chia pudding is a *Fiber Fueled* riff on lemon pudding. Who needs dairy and egg yolks when you have chia seeds? Chia seeds swell when mixed with liquid, creating a thick, creamy pudding out of lemon juice and almond milk. For a creamier pudding, swap in canned coconut milk after Week 3.

Makes about 2 cups

1 cup unsweetened almond milk
1 teaspoon freshly grated lemon zest
¼ cup freshly squeezed lemon juice
1 to 2 tablespoons 100% maple syrup
¼ teaspoon ground turmeric

Pinch salt

¼ cup chia seeds

In a medium bowl, whisk together the almond milk, lemon zest, lemon juice, maple syrup, turmeric, and salt. Add the chia seeds and whisk until very well combined, then place in the fridge for 15 minutes. Remove, whisk together again, then cover and place back in the fridge to gel at least 2 hours, or overnight.

Place in an airtight container and keep in the fridge for up to 7 days.

Make-Ahead Tip:

Make the chia pudding ahead of time. It will keep for up to 1 week in the fridge.

Supercharge It!

Top with berries and up to ½ cup unsweetened shredded coconut. After Week 2, you can add Whipped Coconut Cream (page 253), too.

3 PLANT POINTS

Whipped Coconut Cream

Serves 4

1 can full fat coconut milk (or coconut cream), placed in the fridge overnight

Carefully open the can and scoop out the top half of the solidified coconut. If you are using coconut milk, make sure you are only getting the solid coconut, not the water underneath. You can discard the water or save it for another recipe. If you are using coconut cream, you will use the whole can.

Place the solidified coconut in a bowl and whip until creamy, using a hand mixer or a stand mixer.

1 PLANT POINT

Week 2

One week down! Do you have a favorite recipe so far? How about the Plant Points—did you get Rock Star status already? We're going to keep it pretty gentle in Week 2, but we will introduce some lentils here this week to start exercising the gut a little bit. There are low FODMAP substitutions available if you think you need them. Don't forget about fermented foods! If you're feeling bold, go ahead and add one as a garnish to any recipe that feels right to you and grant yourself an extra Plant Point for your efforts. Make sure to stay connected to our online community by posting your food pictures to #fiberfueled4weeks. Remember, we're all in this together.

WEEK 2 SHOPPING LIST
Produce
- [ ] 1 medium piece fresh ginger
- [ ] 4 large lemons
- [ ] 1 large red bell pepper
- [ ] 1 large green bell pepper
- [ ] 1 ounce dried shiitake mushrooms
- [ ] 1 small onion
- [ ] 1 pound carrots
- [ ] 1 pound celery hearts
- [ ] 1 large baking potato
- [ ] 1 pint cherry tomatoes
- [ ] One 5-ounce bag spinach leaves

- ☐ 1 pound strawberries
- ☐ 3 bananas
- ☐ 1 kiwi
- ☐ One 10-ounce package leafy salad greens
- ☐ 2 beets
- ☐ One 100-gram container broccoli sprouts
- ☐ 1 bunch fresh parsley
- ☐ 1 Thai chili
- ☐ 1 zucchini
- ☐ 1 small bunch fresh chives
- ☐ 3 bunches kale (lacinato or curly)
- ☐ 1 jalapeño
- ☐ 1 bunch fresh cilantro
- ☐ 2 limes
- ☐ 1 bunch fresh mint
- ☐ 1 pint blueberries
- ☐ 3 large sweet potatoes
- ☐ 2 bunches scallions
- ☐ 1 head romaine lettuce
- ☐ 7 large oranges
- ☐ 2 large grapefruit
- ☐ 3 large salad tomatoes
- ☐ 1 small butternut squash
- ☐ One 6-ounce package snow peas
- ☐ 1 small head red cabbage

Cupboard
- ☐ One 24-ounce bag gluten-free flour
- ☐ One 64-ounce container almond milk
- ☐ 4 ounces matcha powder (preferably ceremonial matcha)
- ☐ One 8-ounce bag frozen edamame
- ☐ 8 ounces soba noodles

- ☐ Three 15-ounce cans chickpeas
- ☐ 1 small bag oat flour
- ☐ One 15-ounce can pumpkin puree
- ☐ Pumpkin pie spice
- ☐ Mustard seeds
- ☐ One 1-pound bag dried red lentils
- ☐ One 28-ounce can diced tomatoes
- ☐ One 15-ounce can diced tomatoes
- ☐ Three 15-ounce cans brown lentils
- ☐ 1 loaf sourdough bread
- ☐ Corn tortillas (4)
- ☐ 2 pounds firm tofu, packed in water
- ☐ One 14-ounce package soft tofu
- ☐ One 2.24-ounce can sliced black olives
- ☐ One 8-ounce bag dark chocolate chips or cacao nibs
- ☐ One 8-ounce bag dried cranberries
- ☐ 8 ounces dried goji berries (optional)
- ☐ Two 15-ounce cans coconut milk
- ☐ One 15-ounce can tomato sauce
- ☐ One 8-ounce jar Dijon mustard
- ☐ One 10-ounce bag chopped walnuts
- ☐ 2 pounds chopped frozen spinach

Week 2—Drinks, Snacks, and Dessert

Remember, these recipes are to be enjoyed whenever the moment feels right.

Drink Recipe: Matcha Latte (page 275)

Snack Recipe #1: Pumpkin Hummus (page 276) with cucumbers and carrots

Snack Recipe #2: Plant-Powered Trail Mix (page 277)

Dessert Recipe #1: Chocolate Mousse (page 278)

Dessert Recipe #2: Chickpea Cookie Dough Bites (page 279)

Week 2—Quick-Fix Menu

Quick-Fix Breakfast: Simple Overnight Oats (page 261)

Quick-Fix Lunch: The Daily Salad (page 229) with sourdough toast spread with Pumpkin Hummus (page 276)

Quick-Fix Dinner: No-Tuna Sunflower Salad (page 267) with leftover vegetables and Pumpkin Hummus (page 276)

Quick-Fix Snack: 15 almonds

Quick-Fix Dessert: ⅓ cup blueberries or 15 strawberries

Week 2 Meal Prep

Week 2 Recommended Prep

Red Lentil Curry Soup (page 264)

Chickpea Cookie Dough Bites (page 279)

Pumpkin Hummus (page 276)

Simple Overnight Oats (page 261)

Week 2 Optional Prep

Butternut Squash and Quinoa Chili (page 266)

Slice cucumbers and carrots for a snack on Day 1, then place them in a container with water in the fridge until ready to enjoy with the Pumpkin Hummus (page 276) on Day 2.

Oil-Free Orange Dressing (page 230)

Chocolate Mousse (page 278)

DAY 1 (USUALLY SUNDAY)

Meal	Recipe	Page	Plant Points
Breakfast	Tofu Scramble Bowls with Citrus and Mint Salad	Tofu Scramble: 259 Citrus and mint Salad: 265	3–5

| Lunch | Red Lentil Curry Soup with sourdough bread | 264 | 8 |
| Dinner | Lentil-Walnut Tacos | 269 | 5 |

DAY 2

Meal	Recipe	Page	Plant Points
Breakfast	Pumpkin Pie for Breakfast Smoothie	260	4–5
Lunch	Leftover Mushroom Risotto with Down 'n' Dirty Kale Salad	Mushroom Risotto: 245 Kale Salad: 233	10–12
Dinner	Butternut Squash and Quinoa Chili	266	10–11

DAY 3

Meal	Recipe	Page	Plant Points
Breakfast	Simple Overnight Oats	261	4
Lunch	The Daily Salad with Oil-Free Orange Dressing and leftover Red Lentil Curry Soup	The Daily Salad: 229 soup: 264	17
Dinner	Stuffed Taco Sweet Potatoes	270	6

DAY 4

Meal	Recipe	Page	Plant Points
Breakfast	Superfood Smoothie with nut butter drizzle	225	6
Lunch	Butternut Squash and Quinoa Chili with Down 'n' Dirty Kale Salad	Chili: 266 Kale Salad: 233	15–18
Dinner	Miso, Mushroom, and Soba Bowl	271	9–10

DAY 5

Meal	Recipe	Page	Plant Points
Breakfast	Simple Overnight Oats	261	4
Lunch	The Daily Salad with sourdough toast topped with Pumpkin Hummus	The Daily Salad: 229 Pumpkin Hummus: 276	12–15
Dinner	Saag Tofu	272	5

DAY 6

Meal	Recipe	Page	Plant Points
Breakfast	Super Seedy Breakfast Porridge	223	6
Lunch	Leftover Saag Tofu	272	5
Dinner	Lentil–Sweet Potato Stew	274	7–9

DAY 7

Meal	Recipe	Page	Plant Points
Breakfast	Gluten-Free Pancakes with berries	262	2+
Lunch	No-Tuna Sunflower Salad on sourdough toast with Citrus and Mint Salad	No-Tuna salad: 267 Citrus and Mint Salad: 245	9–10
Dinner	Leftover Lentil–Sweet Potato Stew with Down 'n' Dirty Kale Salad	Lentil Stew: 274 Kale Salad: 233	12–16

BREAKFAST

Tofu Scramble Bowls

Consider this your new favorite brunch. Tofu is lower in saturated fat, lower in monounsaturated fat, and higher in polyunsaturated fats and free of cholesterol compared to eggs, making it the perfect swap.

If you're new to cooking with tofu, know that you'll need to press it first. You can do this with a tofu press, or by wrapping the tofu block in paper towels, placing it on a rimmed baking sheet and placing something heavy on top. Let sit for about 10 minutes to let most of the water drain out. This allows the tofu to become chewier, perfect for egg-like curds.

Serves 2

5 tablespoons vegetable broth

8 ounces firm tofu, drained, pressed, and crumbled or diced

1 scallion, green parts only, sliced

½ teaspoon smoked paprika

½ teaspoon ground turmeric

¼ teaspoon ground cumin

Salt and freshly ground black pepper

2 slices leftover Berry Good Sweet Potato Toast (page 226), cubed

2 cups finely chopped kale, stems removed

Heat a medium skillet over medium heat, add 2 tablespoons vegetable broth, and heat until shimmering. Add the tofu and cook until warmed, about 2 minutes, then add the scallions, paprika, turmeric, cumin, and a pinch of salt. Reduce the heat to low and cook until warmed, stirring occasionally, about 5 more minutes.

In a separate skillet, heat the remaining 3 tablespoons broth over medium heat. Add the sweet potatoes and cook, stirring occasionally, until warm, about 5 minutes. Add the kale and a pinch of salt and pepper and cover. Cook for about 3 minutes, until the greens are just wilted.

Divide the kale and sweet potatoes into two bowls, then top with the tofu mixture. For a heartier meal, add a slice of sourdough toast, with or without peanut or almond butter.

Supercharge It!
Top with chopped parsley, chopped cilantro, and diced tomatoes

3 PLANT POINTS

Pumpkin Pie for Breakfast Smoothie

Pie for breakfast? Sounds good to us! Especially when it's in the form of a sippable, nutrient-dense smoothie, perfect for on-the-go mornings. Serve as is or topped with Crispy Oat Granola (page 228).

Serves 2
2 frozen bananas
1 cup canned coconut milk
1 cup unsweetened almond milk
½ cup pumpkin puree
2 tablespoons maple syrup
2 tablespoons hemp seeds
1 teaspoon pumpkin pie spice
½ teaspoon ground cinnamon
1½ cups ice

Place the bananas, coconut milk, almond milk, pumpkin, maple syrup, hemp seeds, pumpkin pie spice, cinnamon, and ice in a blender and blend until creamy and very smooth.

To make it into a smoothie bowl, reduce the liquid by half (use ½ cup of canned coconut milk and ½ cup of canned almond milk), then blend as directed. Divide the contents into two bowls and add 1 tablespoon pecans and 1 to 2 tablespoons Crispy Oat Granola.

Lower FODMAP Options:

Unripe bananas are lower in FODMAPs than ripe bananas, but you can also reduce this to ½ banana per serving if you are sensitive to fructose. ½ ripe banana or 1 medium unripe banana are both low FODMAPs.

Supercharge It!

Add a handful of fresh or frozen spinach to add an extra boost of vitamins, minerals, and fiber and turn your smoothie green.

4 PLANT POINTS

Simple Overnight Oats

Everyone needs a good overnight oat recipe, and this is our go-to. The beauty of overnight oats is that they are customizable to whatever you are craving: add soy milk for a higher protein breakfast, almond milk for low FODMAP, or coconut milk for a creamier bowl of oats. And get those omega-3s cranking with the super seeds on this one!

Serves 2
⅔ cup old-fashioned oats
1 tablespoon chia seeds
1 tablespoon almond butter or peanut butter
½ teaspoon ground cinnamon
1 cup dairy-free milk of choice or up to 1⅓ cups milk for a thinner oatmeal
¾ cup fruit of choice
Maple syrup, if desired

In a resealable jar or bowl, combine the oats, chia seeds, nut butter, and cinnamon. Add a splash of the milk and mix everything together, working the nut butter into the oats as much as possible. Add the rest of the milk and stir to combine.

Cover the bowl or place the lid on the jar and refrigerate, up to 4 days. When ready to serve, mix in the fruit and a drizzle of maple syrup, if desired.

Low FODMAP Options:

Lower FODMAP fruit options include raspberries, blueberries, strawberries, pineapple, kiwi, and papaya.

Supercharge It!

Add in hemp seeds, additional chia seeds, fruit (especially berries), and unsweetened shredded coconut.

4 PLANT POINTS

Gluten-Free Pancakes

Three cheers for pancakes! These gluten-free pancakes are perfect for lazy weekend mornings. Serve them plain, or as berry pancakes by mixing fresh chopped fruit into the finished batter.

Makes 6 pancakes

1 tablespoon ground flaxseed

3 tablespoons water

1 cup gluten-free flour

1 teaspoon baking powder

¼ teaspoon baking soda

¼ teaspoon salt

1 cup unsweetened almond milk

1 teaspoon apple cider vinegar

1 tablespoon organic sunflower oil, plus more for greasing the skillet
1 tablespoon vanilla extract

Whisk together the flaxseed and 3 tablespoons water and set aside until jelled, about 5 minutes.

In a large mixing bowl, whisk together the gluten-free flour, baking powder, baking soda, and salt in a large mixing bowl. Set aside.

In a separate medium bowl, add the almond milk and vinegar. Then add in the sunflower oil, vanilla, and the jelled flax. Whisk to incorporate, then add the almond milk mixture into the flour mixture and whisk thoroughly until no lumps remain.

Grease and heat a large skillet with coconut oil or cooking spray over medium-high heat. Drop batter into the hot skillet, using a ¼ cup measuring cup. Wait for large bubbles to form, then flip and cook another 60 seconds, until golden brown on both sides.

Serve with berries and maple syrup, if desired.

Supercharge It!
Add chopped berries to the batter.

2 PLANT POINTS

LUNCH

Red Lentil Curry Soup

There is nothing more soothing than sipping on an incredibly nourishing soup loaded with vegetables, lentils, and spices. After a bowl of this, we're ready to conquer the world! Well, at least conquer our to-do list. For a heartier meal, serve with Down 'n' Dirty Kale Salad (page 233) or toasted sourdough bread.

Serves 4, with leftovers for later in the week

1 tablespoon garlic-infused olive oil (see page 246)

¼ cup finely chopped onion

1 celery stalk, chopped

3 large carrots, chopped

1 large baking potato, chopped

1 teaspoon ground cumin

1 teaspoon ground turmeric

1 teaspoon smoked paprika

½ teaspoon ground ginger

½ teaspoon curry powder

½ teaspoon salt, plus more to taste

½ teaspoon freshly ground black pepper, plus more to taste

4 cups vegetable broth or Biome Broth (page 249)

1¼ cups red lentils

One 28-ounce can diced tomatoes, drained

½ cup chopped fresh parsley or fresh cilantro

1 tablespoon freshly squeezed lemon juice

Heat the olive oil in a large saucepan over medium heat. Add the onion and let cook until soft, 5 to 7 minutes.

Add the celery, carrots, and potato. Cook until soft and lightly browned, another 10 minutes. Add the cumin, turmeric, paprika, ginger, curry powder, salt, and pepper then stir until fragrant, 30 to 60 seconds.

Add the broth, lentils, and tomatoes and bring to a simmer. Cover and cook for 20 minutes, or until the lentils are tender. Remove from the heat, let cool slightly, then puree half of the soup either using a blender or immersion blender. Add the pureed soup back into the pot, then stir in the herbs and lemon juice. Add salt and pepper to taste.

Low FODMAP Options:

Onions have moderate GOS. Replace with ¼ cup fresh or dried chives at the same time as the celery, carrots, and chopped potato.

Red lentils have moderate GOS. Reduce the amount used to 1 cup so that only ¼ cup cooked is in each serving.

8 PLANT POINTS

Citrus and Mint Salad

This refreshing salad is one of our favorite lettuce-free options. Great as a side dish, dessert, or simple snack. We've called for orange and grapefruit here, but it can be subbed with any citrus. As someone who grew up in Syracuse, New York, I'm required to say "Let's Go Orange!"

Serves 2

2 large oranges, peeled, pith removed, and segmented
1 large grapefruit, peeled, pith removed, and segmented* *yellow light, fructan for ½ cup serving*
Zest and juice of 1 lime
1 teaspoon 100% maple syrup
1 tablespoon minced fresh mint

Toss together the segmented oranges and grapefruit with the lime zest, juice, and maple syrup. Divide between two plates and sprinkle with the fresh mint.

Low FODMAP Option:

Grapefruits have moderate fructans. Reduce the amount of grapefruit in this recipe to ½ grapefruit (¼ grapefruit per serving), which is low FODMAP.

3 PLANT POINTS

Butternut Squash and Quinoa Chili

This butternut squash and quinoa chili is a thick, soul-warming dish packed with vegetables.

Makes 2 servings

1¼ cups Biome Broth (page 249)

⅔ cup peeled and diced butternut squash

¼ cup sliced scallions, green parts only

¼ medium green bell pepper, diced

¼ medium red bell pepper, diced

½ jalapeño, seeds and ribs removed, finely diced

1 cup (8 ounces) canned diced tomatoes

1 large carrot, diced

½ medium zucchini, diced

1½ teaspoons smoked paprika

1 teaspoon ground cumin

Salt and freshly ground black pepper

1 cup cooked quinoa

Heat 1 tablespoon of broth in a large saucepan over medium heat. Add the butternut squash and cook, stirring often and adding more broth as needed to prevent the squash from sticking, until just softened, stirring often, 5 to 8 minutes.

Add the scallions, bell peppers, and jalapeño and cook, stirring occasionally, for an additional 5 minutes. Add another tablespoon of the broth to prevent sticking, if necessary.

Add the diced tomatoes, carrot, zucchini, paprika, cumin, and remaining broth.

Bring the mixture to a boil, then cover and reduce the heat to low and simmer for 15 minutes, until the vegetables are soft.

Taste and adjust the seasonings as needed, adding salt and pepper to taste. Add the cooked quinoa and allow to cook for about 5 more minutes. Serve.

Low FODMAP Option:

Some canned tomatoes contain garlic and onion. Check the ingredient list.

Make-Ahead Tips:

This dish requires cooked quinoa, so cooking the quinoa ahead of time will make for easier meal prep.

Supercharge It!

Top with fresh herbs, like parsley.

10 PLANT POINTS

No-Tuna Sunflower Salad

Sunflower seeds take the place of tuna in this twist on a classic. The lemon, parsley, and chives give this salad a bright flavor, and pulsing all the ingredients in the food processor creates a similar texture to that other tuna salad.

Makes 4 servings, with enough for leftovers later in the week

1 cup sunflower seeds

Juice of 2 large lemons

1 tablespoon Dijon mustard

½ cup roughly chopped fresh parsley, stems removed

½ cup roughly chopped fresh chives

¼ teaspoon smoked paprika

2 celery stalks, chopped

4 scallions, green parts only, chopped

½ teaspoon salt

Pinch freshly ground black pepper

8 slices of sourdough bread, for serving

Salad greens, for serving

Sliced tomato, for serving

Place the sunflower seeds in a sealable container and cover with water. Soak at room temperature for at least 24 hours. They should double in size. When ready to use, drain the water off the seeds, add fresh water to cover, then drain again.

Place ½ cup of sunflower seeds into the base of a food processor along with the lemon juice and mustard. Pulse 10 times, until finely chopped.

Add the remaining ½ cup sunflower seeds, the parsley, chives, paprika, celery, scallions, salt, and black pepper. Pulse in a food processor until the texture is similar to traditional tuna salad, about 10 more times.

Serve on toasted sourdough bread, with salad greens and sliced tomato.

Make-Ahead Options:
Prep the sunflower seeds at least one day ahead of making this salad.

Supercharge It!
Toss 1 teaspoon of chia seeds into this salad for extra crunch, healthy fats, and plant points!

6 PLANT POINTS

DINNER

Lentil-Walnut Tacos

You'll use this lentil walnut taco filling in both the Lentil Walnut
Tacos and the Stuffed Taco Sweet Potatoes. We love recipes that do
double duty and save you time in the kitchen.

*Makes 4 servings, with enough for leftovers for Stuffed Taco
Sweet Potatoes*

½ cup walnuts, finely chopped

1 tablespoon olive oil or Biome Broth (page 249)

1 large tomato, chopped

Two 14.5-ounce cans brown lentils, drained and rinsed

2 teaspoons dried oregano

2 teaspoons ground cumin

2 tablespoons chili powder

½ teaspoon salt

¼ cup water

Tacos

4 to 6 corn tortillas

½ recipe Lentil Walnut Filling

Creamy Cilantro Sauce (page 237), for serving

Diced tomatoes, chopped fresh cilantro, shredded lettuce, and/or
sliced black olives, for serving

Stuffed Taco Sweet Potatoes

2 medium sweet potatoes

½ recipe Lentil Walnut Filling

Creamy Cilantro Sauce (page 237)

Diced tomatoes, chopped fresh cilantro, shredded lettuce, and/or
sliced black olives, for serving

Heat a large skillet over medium heat and add the walnuts. Toast, stirring often, for about 2 minutes, until the walnuts are lightly browned and fragrant, taking care not to burn. Remove the walnuts from the skillet and set aside.

Add the oil and tomato to the same skillet and cook until the tomato is soft, 3 to 4 more minutes. Add the canned lentils, oregano, cumin, chili powder, salt, and water. Cook until heated through, gently mashing some of the lentils with the back of a wooden spoon or spatula, for 5 minutes.

Taste, adding more chili powder or salt, if desired.

To make the tacos: Warm the corn tortillas and top with the filling and the toppings of your choice.

To make the stuffed sweet potatoes: Preheat the oven to 400°F. Using a fork, poke the sweet potatoes a few times on each side to help release steam as they cook. Place directly into the oven and cook until tender, 45 to 55 minutes for smaller sweet potatoes, 55 to 70 minutes for larger ones.

Remove the potatoes from the oven and split them down the middle. Top with the Lentil-Walnut Filling, Creamy Cilantro Sauce, and desired toppings.

TACOS—5 PLANT POINTS

STUFFED SWEET POTATOES—6 PLANT POINTS

Lower FODMAP Option:

½ cup serving of canned, cooked lentils is considered low FODMAP. A larger serving has moderate GOS. If you are sensitive to this food, pay close attention to portion size.

Chili powder can contain garlic and onion. Garlic is high in FODMAPs (fructan) and onion is high in fructan and has moderate amounts of GOS. If you find that you are sensitive to either of these, substitute smoked paprika here.

Miso, Mushroom, and Soba Bowl

"Soba" is the Japanese word for "buckwheat," which is the wheat-free flour that makes up soba noodles. *Oishi* is the Japanese word for "delicious," which is what you'll be saying while you enjoy the soba.

Makes 2 bowls

½ cup frozen, shelled edamame

4 ounces uncooked soba noodles

10 to 20 snow peas, vertically sliced

2 teaspoons sesame oil

¼ cup Biome Broth (page 249) or vegetable broth

1 teaspoon miso paste

¼ teaspoon 100% maple syrup

1 teaspoon grated fresh ginger

¼ teaspoon salt, plus more to taste

1 teaspoon garlic-infused olive oil (see page 246)

1 cup thinly sliced red cabbage

4 rehydrated dried shiitake mushrooms, stems removed and sliced

1 to 2 carrots, shaved into ribbons with vegetable peeler (1 large or 2 small)

4 scallions (green parts only), sliced

Bring a medium saucepan of water to boil over medium-high heat. Add the edamame and soba noodles and cook for 2 minutes.

Add in the sliced snow peas and cook for an additional minute, until the noodles are tender. Drain and rinse with cold water to stop cooking. Set aside.

In a small bowl, whisk together the sesame oil, broth, miso paste, maple syrup, ginger, and salt. Set aside.

Heat the olive oil in a medium skillet over medium heat, then add in the cabbage, mushrooms, carrots, and scallions. Toss and cook for about 3 minutes, until just tender.

Add the edamame, noodles, snow peas, and sesame sauce to the skillet and toss until the dish is heated through, 2 to 3 minutes.

Lower FODMAP Options:

5 snowpea pods per serving is considered low FODMAP, while 7 snowpea pods is considered moderate FODMAP (fructan and mannitol).

2 shiitake mushrooms per serving is considered low FODMAP. Feel free to increase the serving here if you are not sensitive to mannitol.

Supercharge It!

Add a serving of cooked tofu for a higher protein dish.

Make-Ahead Tip:

Prep the sauce and chop the vegetables ahead of time, then store in the fridge until ready to use.

9 PLANT POINTS

Saag Tofu

We hope you love Indian food as much as we do, because we cannot get enough! While we're partial to almost any vegetable in a fragrant curry sauce, saag tofu is one of our favorites. The ingredient list seems long, but rest assured that it's mostly spices. If these spices are new to you, consider purchasing them from the bulk section of your grocery store so you're able to get only a tablespoon or two of what you need.

Serves 4, with enough for leftovers for later in the week
2 teaspoons garlic-infused olive oil (see page 246)
2 tablespoons freshly grated ginger
1 Thai chile, seeded and chopped
1½ tablespoons garam masala

1 tablespoon ground coriander

1 tablespoon ground turmeric

1 tablespoon ground cumin

½ teaspoon ground cayenne pepper

1 teaspoon mustard seeds

1 teaspoon salt, plus more as needed

2 pounds frozen chopped spinach (5 cups), thawed and drained

1 cup canned full-fat coconut milk

1 cup tomato sauce

One 14-ounce package firm or extra-firm tofu, drained and pressed

2 teaspoons cornstarch

Freshly ground black pepper

2 cups cooked rice, to serve

Heat 1 teaspoon olive oil in a medium skillet over medium heat. Stir in the ginger, chili, garam masala, coriander, turmeric, cumin, cayenne, mustard seeds, and salt. Cook for another 30 to 60 seconds, until just fragrant.

Add the spinach leaves to the skillet and cook to wilt, 1 to 2 minutes. Remove from the heat and let cool slightly.

Add the spinach to the base of a food processor and pulse to finely chop the mixture. Add back to the skillet along with the coconut milk and tomato sauce, then let simmer, stirring occasionally, for 30 minutes.

While the spinach is simmering, make the tofu. Dice the tofu and toss with the cornstarch in a medium bowl until well-coated. Heat the remaining teaspoon of olive oil in a large skillet over medium heat, then add in the tofu. Cook, stirring often, until the tofu is golden brown and crispy. Add the cooked tofu to the spinach mixture and stir to combine.

Season to taste, adding in more salt and pepper as needed and serve warm with cooked rice.

Low FODMAP Options:

More than 2¾ cups spinach has moderate fructans.

5 PLANT POINTS

Lentil–Sweet Potato Stew

Garlic-infused olive oil and fresh ginger really make the curry stand out! Make a batch of this soup on the weekend and reheat for lunches or dinner during a busy week.

Serves 2

1 teaspoon garlic-infused olive oil (see page 246)

1 teaspoon minced fresh ginger

1 carrot, chopped

Salt and freshly ground black pepper

2 tablespoon dried or fresh chives (finely chopped if fresh)

1 sweet potato, peeled and chopped

2 teaspoons curry powder, plus more to taste

2½ cups Biome Broth (page 249) or vegetable broth

½ cup canned lentils

1 large handful fresh spinach or kale leaves

Heat a medium pot over medium heat. Add the olive oil, ginger, and chopped carrots. Sprinkle with a pinch of salt and pepper, then cook for 3 minutes, stirring occasionally.

Add the chives and sweet potato and cook for an additional 5 minutes, stirring occasionally. Stir in the curry powder.

Add the broth to the pot, cover, and raise the heat to medium-high to bring to a low boil. Add the lentils to the soup and stir to combine. Reduce the heat to low and simmer, uncovered, for about 20 minutes, until the potatoes are fork tender.

Add salt, pepper, or curry powder to taste. Just before serving, stir in the greens until just wilted. Serve with a side of sourdough bread, if preferred.

Make-Ahead Tips:
Chop the sweet potato and carrot ahead of time.

Supercharge It!
Top with fresh scallions and parsley.

7 PLANT POINTS

SNACKS, DRINKS, AND DESSERTS

Matcha Latte

This antioxidant-rich beverage is the perfect pick-me-up. We recommend almond milk for Week 1, with the option of choosing soy milk after Week 2 for higher protein. After Week 3, you can also use coconut milk for a creamier latte. Whatever dairy-free milk you prefer, we recommend one without carrageenan.

Serves 2
1½ cups unsweetened almond milk
2 teaspoons matcha powder (organic ceremonial matcha powder will have better flavor than culinary matcha)
½ cup boiling water
100% maple syrup, as desired, to taste

Bring the almond milk to a low simmer in a small pot over medium-high heat.

Place 1 teaspoon matcha powder at the bottom of two mugs. Slowly whisk ¼ cup boiling water into each mug, completely dissolving the matcha powder. Keep whisking, then add the warm milk, tipping the cup slightly to help create more foam. Sweeten with maple syrup, if desired.

For an iced latte, whisk the matcha powder with enough water to form a paste, stirring so there are no clumps. Add cold unsweetened almond milk and stir vigorously until well mixed. Divide between two glasses, stir in the maple syrup, as desired, and serve over ice.

2 PLANT POINTS

Pumpkin Hummus

Pumpkin is a fantastic source of fiber, vitamin A, and antioxidants. This savory pumpkin dip tastes wonderful with fresh vegetables, whole-grain sourdough toast, or any other way you can think to use it!

Makes 2 cups
One 15-ounce can chickpeas, drained and rinsed
⅔ cup pumpkin puree
½ teaspoon salt
1 teaspoon ground cumin
Juice of ½ large lemon
1 tablespoon garlic-infused olive oil (see page 246)

Place the chickpeas, pumpkin, salt, cumin, lemon juice, and olive oil in the base of a food processor. Blend until smooth and creamy, scraping down the sides as needed.

Transfer to an airtight container and store in the fridge for up to 1 week.

Lower FODMAP Options:

Enjoy a smaller, 2-tablespoon serving of the hummus for a lower FODMAP option.

Supercharge It!

Sprinkle the hummus with pumpkin seeds or hemp seeds for extra protein, healthy fats, crunch, and Plant Points.

3 PLANT POINTS

Plant-Powered Trail Mix

This snack mix will keep you powered throughout the day with fiber and plant-based protein.

Makes 2 servings
2 tablespoons pepitas
2 tablespoons almonds
2 tablespoons walnuts
2 tablespoons dark chocolate chips or cacao nibs
2 tablespoons dried cranberries

Combine the pepitas, almonds, walnuts, chocolate chips, and cranberries in an airtight container or bag and store until ready to eat.

Supercharge It!

Add 1 tablespoon goji berries.

4 PLANT POINTS

Chocolate Mousse

Creamy, sweet, and perfectly satisfying, this chocolate mousse is a plant protein–packed sweet treat.

Note: Place the can of coconut milk in the refrigerator upside down for at least 3 hours. This will allow the coconut milk fat/solids to harden and separate from the liquid. This helps make the mousse creamier!

Serves 4 to 6
1 block soft tofu, drained but not pressed
½ cup canned coconut milk
½ cup 100% maple syrup
½ cup unsweetened cocoa powder
2 tablespoons peanut butter
1 teaspoon vanilla extract
1 teaspoon salt

Place the tofu, coconut milk, maple syrup, cocoa powder, peanut butter, vanilla, and salt into the base of a food processor or high-powered blender. Puree until very smooth, scraping down the sides as necessary.

Divide among 4 to 6 ramekins or small bowls and allow to chill in the refrigerator for 30 minutes or more to set.

Supercharge It!
Add up to 30 raspberries per serving for added sweet flavor, fiber, and another Plant Point.

Low FODMAP Options:
Silken tofu is high FODMAP, but firm tofu is not high FODMAP in a ⅔-cup serving size.

3 PLANT POINTS

Chickpea Cookie Dough Bites

Cookie dough, but it's healthy? Yep. We play to win the game. If you don't have oat flour, place ½ cup rolled oats in a blender or food processor and process until a fine flour forms.

Makes about 16 balls

One 15-ounce can chickpeas, drained, rinsed, and pat dry

⅓ cup oat flour

¼ cup peanut butter

3 tablespoons 100% maple syrup, plus more as desired

1 teaspoon vanilla extract

¼ teaspoon salt

¼ teaspoon ground cinnamon

⅓ cup dairy-free chocolate chips (Enjoy Life Foods has many low FODMAP–certified products, including chocolate chips!)

Place the chickpeas, oat flour, peanut butter, maple syrup, vanilla, salt, and cinnamon in the base of a food processor.

Process until a dough forms. Taste, adding in more maple syrup as desired.

Fold in the chocolate chips, then pulse until just combined and the chips are incorporated.

Roll into balls and place on a parchment paper–lined rimmed baking sheet. Store in the fridge to harden for at least 15 minutes. Transfer to an airtight container and keep in the fridge for up to 1 week.

Make-Ahead Tips:

Make ahead of time for quick snacks throughout the week.

2 PLANT POINTS

Week 3

More than halfway done! You're making great progress. So now that
we're two weeks in, we're going to start ramping things up a little bit.
This week you'll be seeing some garlic, onions, and grains. I love these
flavors and know they will excite your taste buds. Don't forget to drink
the Lemon Ginger Tea if the mood hits you. You'll also see some famil-
iar recipes from Week 1 that will make a guest appearance here in Week
3. Make sure to use the low FODMAP recipe options when you think
it's necessary. And as always, post your experience to #fiberfueled4weeks
so I can follow your progress and so we can all be in it together as a
community.

WEEK 3 SHOPPING LIST

Produce

- ☐ 1 medium piece fresh ginger
- ☐ 5 large lemons
- ☐ 3 large red bell peppers
- ☐ 1 yellow bell pepper
- ☐ 2 large green bell peppers
- ☐ 1 ounce dried shiitake mushrooms
- ☐ 2 medium yellow or white onions
- ☐ 1 pound carrots
- ☐ 1 pound celery hearts
- ☐ 4 large cucumbers
- ☐ 1 pint cherry tomatoes
- ☐ 1 5-ounce bag spinach leaves
- ☐ 6 bananas
- ☐ 4 kiwis
- ☐ 1 5-ounce package leafy salad greens
- ☐ 1 100-gram container broccoli sprouts
- ☐ 1 bunch fresh parsley

- ☐ 3 large avocados
- ☐ 1 bunch fresh chives
- ☐ 1 Roma tomato
- ☐ 1 bunch kale (lacinato or curly)
- ☐ 1 jalapeño
- ☐ 3 bunches fresh cilantro
- ☐ 6 limes
- ☐ 1 large spaghetti squash
- ☐ 1 shallot
- ☐ 1 head garlic
- ☐ 16 ounces peanuts
- ☐ 2 honeydew melons
- ☐ 1 bunch fresh mint
- ☐ 2 pints berries of choice
- ☐ 1 large sweet potato
- ☐ 3 bunches scallions
- ☐ 1 head romaine lettuce
- ☐ 2 bunches baby bok choy
- ☐ 4 ounces shiitake mushrooms
- ☐ 2 teaspoons tomato paste
- ☐ 1 pound dried brown lentils
- ☐ ¼ cup raw cashews
- ☐ 1 large tomato
- ☐ 1 small head red or green Napa cabbage
- ☐ 4 collard leaves
- ☐ 1 medium onion
- ☐ 1 bunch asparagus

Cupboard

- ☐ One 64-ounce container almond milk
- ☐ One 8-ounce bag frozen edamame in pods

- ☐ One 16-ounce bag rolled oats
- ☐ One 2-ounce bag sliced almonds
- ☐ One 8-ounce bag frozen cherries
- ☐ 2 ounces mushroom powder
- ☐ 8 ounces soba noodles
- ☐ Three 15-ounce cans chickpeas
- ☐ One 4-ounce jar kalamata olives
- ☐ One 8-ounce jar Dijon mustard
- ☐ One 12-ounce bag frozen okra
- ☐ One 14-ounce can kidney beans
- ☐ One 16-ounce jar kimchi
- ☐ One 8-ounce bag farro
- ☐ One 15-ounce can pumpkin puree
- ☐ One 15-ounce can black beans
- ☐ One 16-package red lentils
- ☐ One 15-ounce can fire-roasted diced tomatoes
- ☐ 1 loaf sourdough bread
- ☐ Corn tortillas (4)
- ☐ 4 pounds extra-firm tofu, packed in water
- ☐ Capers
- ☐ One 2.24-ounce can sliced black olives
- ☐ One 15-ounce can tomato sauce
- ☐ One 32-ounce container vegetable broth
- ☐ Vegan Worcestershire sauce
- ☐ 1 small jar hot sauce, like Texas Pete

Week 3—Drinks, Snacks, and Dessert

Remember, these recipes are to be enjoyed whenever the moment feels right.

Drink Recipe: The Green Drink (page 309)

Snack Recipe #1: Speedy Edamame (page 310)

Snack Recipe #2: Turmeric Energy Bites (page 310)

Dessert Recipe #1: Chocolate Banana Nice Cream (page 312)

Dessert Recipe #2: Mushroom Hot Cocoa (page 312)

Week 3—Quick-Fix Menu

Quick-Fix Breakfast: Chocolate Peanut Butter Super Smoothie (page 287)

Quick-Fix Lunch: Mediterranean Grain Salad (page 291)

Quick-Fix Dinner: Wild Biome Super Soup (page 232)

Quick-Fix Snack: 20 almonds

Quick-Fix Dessert: 1 cup blueberries or 20 strawberries

Week 3 Meal Prep

Week 3 Recommended Prep

Biome Broth (page 249)

Sesame Noodle Meal Prep Bowl (page 292)

Make both the Crispy Baked Tofu (page 294) and the Sesame
 Dressing from the Sesame Noodle Meal Prep Bowl (page 292)

Simple Overnight Oats (page 261)

Mediterranean Grain Salad (page 291)

Turmeric Energy Bites (page 310)

Week 3 Optional Prep

Berry Good Sweet Potato Toast ahead of time, then toast right before serving for breakfast on Day 6.

Make the Gumbo on Day 1, then place half in the fridge for dinner on Day 4 and the remaining half in the freezer for dinner on Day 4 in Week 4.

Prep the vegetables on Day 1 for the Thai Rainbow Bowls with Peanut Tofu on Day 2.

DAY 1 (USUALLY SUNDAY)

Meal	Recipe	Page	Plant Points
Breakfast	Puttanesca Tofu Scramble with Matcha Latte	Tofu Scramble: 286 Latte: 275	9
Lunch	Colorful Collard Wraps	289	9
Dinner	Lentil Bolognese with Spaghetti Squash and Down 'n' Dirty Kale Salad and Pepita Parmesan	Lentil Bolognese: 297 Kale Salad: 233 Pepita Parmesan: 301	12–17

DAY 2

Meal	Recipe	Page	Plant Points
Breakfast	Superfood Smoothie Bowl	225	6
Lunch	Leftover No-Tuna Sunflower Salad on sourdough	267	7
Dinner	Thai Rainbow Bowls with Peanut Tofu	297	10

DAY 3

Meal	Recipe	Page	Plant Points
Breakfast	Simple Overnight Oats	261	4
Lunch	Sesame Noodle Meal Prep Bowl	292	10
Dinner	Buffalo Chickpea Salad	301	7

DAY 4

Meal	Recipe	Page	Plant Points
Breakfast	Chocolate Peanut Butter Super Smoothie	287	4
Lunch	Mediterranean Grain Salad	291	8
Dinner	Gumbo	303	7

DAY 5

Meal	Recipe	Page	Plant Points
Breakfast	Simple Overnight Oats	261	4
Lunch	Sesame Noodle Meal Prep Bowl	292	10
Dinner	Buffalo Chickpea Salad	301	7

DAY 6

Meal	Recipe	Page	Plant Points
Breakfast	Berry Good Sweet Potato Toast	226	3
Lunch	Mediterranean Grain Salad	291	8
Dinner	Kimchi Fried Rice	305	7

DAY 7

Meal	Recipe	Page	Plant Points
Breakfast	Spicy Breakfast Tacos	288	6
Lunch	Nourishing Buddha Bowl	295	6
Dinner	Lentil Masala	307	6

BREAKFAST

Puttanesca Tofu Scramble

We took our favorite pasta sauce and turned it into a breakfast scramble. Because why would you not!

Serves 2
1 tablespoon vegetable broth or Biome Broth (page 249)
1 tablespoon olive oil
1 scallion (green parts only), thinly sliced
1 Roma tomato, chopped
¼ teaspoon crushed red pepper flakes, plus more to taste (optional)
½ teaspoon dried thyme
½ teaspoon dried oregano
8 ounces extra-firm tofu, drained and pressed
¼ teaspoon ground turmeric
Salt
1 tablespoon capers, drained
¼ cup sliced black olives
Freshly ground black pepper
Fresh parsley, chopped, for serving

In a large skillet over medium heat, combine the vegetable broth and olive oil. Add the scallion, tomato, red pepper flakes (if using), thyme, and oregano. Sauté for about 5 minutes, until the vegetables are softened.

Use a spatula to move the veggies to one side of the pan, then crumble in the tofu, gently breaking the tofu up into small curds so that it resembles eggs. Add the turmeric and a pinch of salt, then cook for 2 to 3 minutes, stirring often, until the tofu is warmed through.

Add the capers and black olives and toss together. Add salt, black pepper, and red pepper flakes to taste. Top with fresh parsley. Serve as is or with toasted sourdough.

7 PLANT POINTS

Chocolate Peanut Butter Super Smoothie

This super smoothie is so thick and creamy, you might mistake it for a milk shake! Packed with plant-based protein and satisfying healthy fats, this super smoothie will keep you full for hours.

Makes 2 smoothies
2 frozen bananas
¼ cup cocoa powder
¼ cup peanut butter
2 tablespoons hemp seeds
3 cups almond or soy milk
2 teaspoons 100% maple syrup or 1 date
Handful of ice cubes

Combine the bananas, cocoa powder, peanut butter, hemp seeds, almond milk, maple syrup, and a handful of ice cubes in a blender and puree until creamy and smooth. Divide into two glasses and serve.

To make it into a smoothie bowl, reduce the milk to ¾ cup and top it with your favorite toppers. We love a few extra slices of banana, our Crispy Oat Granola (page 228), and a drizzle of peanut butter.

Lower FODMAP Options:
Unripe bananas are lower in FODMAPs than ripe bananas. Half a ripe banana or 1 medium unripe banana are both low FODMAP. Use ½ banana per serving if you are sensitive to fructose. Dates are higher in fructans, so use maple syrup if necessary.

Supercharge It!

Add 1 teaspoon of chia seeds for an extra dose of healthy fats.

4 PLANT POINTS

Spicy Breakfast Tacos

Tacos for breakfast? Yes, please! Feel free to adjust the spice by decreasing the amount of jalapeño used in the salsa.

Makes 4 tacos

Cherry Tomato Salsa

¼ cup sliced cherry tomatoes

½ jalapeño, seeded and sliced

2 teaspoons garlic-infused olive oil (see page 246)

1 garlic clove, minced

Juice of ½ lime (save the other half for serving)

Pinch salt

Pinch freshly ground black pepper

Spicy Tofu Taco Filling

½ cup black beans

¾ teaspoon smoked paprika

¾ teaspoon ground cumin

2 teaspoons fresh chopped chives

Dash cayenne pepper (optional)

¼ teaspoon salt

¼ teaspoon freshly ground black pepper

1 teaspoon olive oil

6 ounces firm tofu, drained, rinsed, and pressed

4 corn tortillas

¼ cup fresh cilantro

¼ avocado, sliced

Make the salsa: In a small bowl, combine the sliced cherry tomatoes, jalapeño, olive oil, garlic, and lime juice with a pinch of salt and pepper. Set aside.

Make the taco filling: In a small saucepan, heat the black beans along with 2 tablespoons of water, ¼ teaspoon smoked paprika, ½ teaspoon cumin, 1 teaspoon chives, and a small pinch of cayenne, if using. Continue to cook for about 5 minutes, until warm. Gently smash the mixture using the back of a spoon, leaving some black beans whole. Set aside.

In a small bowl, add the remaining ½ teaspoon paprika, ½ teaspoon cumin, 1 teaspoon chives, dash cayenne, if using, and salt and pepper. Add 2 tablespoons water and whisk together. Set aside.

Heat the oil in a medium skillet over medium heat. Once hot, crumble the drained tofu into the pan along with the reserved taco sauce. Cook, stirring occasionally, for 5 minutes, or until heated through and the seasoning is absorbed.

To serve, warm the tortillas in a clean and dry skillet until warm and flexible. Top with the tofu, black beans, cilantro, avocado, cherry tomato salsa, and a squeeze of fresh lime juice. Serve warm.

Low FODMAP Options:

Garlic is high in fructans. Sub garlic-infused olive oil for the regular olive oil if you're sensitive.

Black beans have moderate GOS. Sub ¼ cup chickpeas.

6 PLANT POINTS

LUNCH

Colorful Collard Wraps

Collard greens are rich in vitamin A, vitamin K, and calcium. Incredibly nutrient-dense and wildly underrated, they're not just for

Southern cooking! Filling these greens with flavorful goodies makes a perfect midday meal.

Makes 4 collard wraps

6 ounces firm or extra-firm tofu, drained and pressed

1 tablespoon tamari

1 teaspoon garlic-infused olive oil (see page 246)

4 collard leaves

½ cup Pumpkin Hummus (page 276)

½ cup red or yellow bell pepper strips

½ cup thinly sliced red cabbage

1 carrot, sliced into short, thin strips

½ cup sliced cucumber (short, thin strips)

½ avocado

2 tablespoons hemp seeds

Preheat the oven to 400°F. Line a large rimmed baking sheet with parchment paper (or lightly spray with cooking oil) and set aside.

Slice the tofu into rectangles or strips, then toss with the tamari and olive oil. Place the tofu on the prepared baking sheet and bake for 30 minutes, flipping halfway through. Remove from the oven and set aside.

Wash and dry the collard leaves, then use a small paring knife to shave the stem to be flush to the leaf so it's easier to roll.

Place the collard leaves on a flat surface and spread 2 tablespoons of the hummus on each leaf near the top/middle of the leaf.

Divide the pepper, cabbage, carrot, cucumber, and avocado among the 4 leaves, then sprinkle with the hemp seeds.

Wrap like a burrito, then slice in half and serve.

Supercharge It!

Add broccoli sprouts.

9 PLANT POINTS

Mediterranean Grain Salad

This grain salad is perfect for lunch or easy dinners. Mix all of the ingredients together, then toss with the dressing right before serving. To pack for work, assemble the salad without the dressing in one container and the dressing in another. Toss together, then enjoy.

Makes 6 cups
Mediterranean Grain Salad
1 cup uncooked farro
1 cup chickpeas
1 large tomato, diced
1 medium red bell pepper, chopped
1 medium yellow bell pepper, chopped
½ cup seeded and chopped cucumber
¼ cup sliced kalamata olives
¼ cup chopped fresh parsley
Zesty Lemon Dressing
1 teaspoon freshly grated lemon zest
¼ cup freshly squeezed lemon juice
1 medium garlic clove, minced
1 teaspoon Dijon mustard
Salt and freshly ground black pepper
3 tablespoons olive oil

Make the grain salad: Bring 3 cups water to a boil in a medium saucepan over medium-high heat and add the farro. Cover, reduce the heat to medium-low, and simmer for 25 to 30 minutes, until the farro is tender. Drain and rinse under cold water and set aside.

Combine the cooked farro, chickpeas, tomato, red and yellow bell peppers, cucumber, olives, and parsley in a large bowl and toss together. Set aside.

Make the dressing: In a separate small bowl, whisk together the lemon zest, lemon juice, garlic, Dijon, and a generous pinch of salt and pepper until well combined, then slowly drizzle in the olive oil.

Assemble: Toss the dressing with the grain salad until well combined, adding more salt and pepper as desired. Store in the fridge. Leftovers will keep for 2 to 3 days in the fridge.

Low FODMAP Options:

Farro is high in fructans. Millet, quinoa, and brown rice are lower FODMAP options.

Chickpeas have moderate GOS. Reduce to ½ cup.

Garlic is high in fructans. Omit and use 1 teaspoon garlic-infused olive oil (see page 246) instead.

Make-Ahead Tips:

Cook the farro ahead of time; it will keep for up to 5 or 6 days in the fridge. Combine the farro with other vegetables and place in an airtight container in the fridge. Make the dressing and place in a resealable airtight jar in the fridge. Toss together before serving.

8 PLANT POINTS

Sesame Noodle Meal Prep Bowl

These cold, Asian-inspired noodles are part of the Sunday meal-prep routine to be used for lunch later in the week. But if you start drooling when you prep them, we won't hold it against you if you give them a little taste.

Makes 4 bowls

Sesame Dressing

¼ cup tahini paste

2 tablespoons warm water

1 tablespoon tamari

2 teaspoons toasted sesame oil

Juice of 1 lime

½ teaspoon minced garlic

½ teaspoon 100% maple syrup

¼ teaspoon crushed red pepper flakes (optional)

Sesame Noodle Bowls

8 ounces soba noodles

2 cups frozen shelled edamame, thawed

2 medium carrots, sliced very thin

2 cups diced cucumber

1 recipe Crispy Baked Tofu (page 294)

2 tablespoons sesame seeds, for serving

2 tablespoons hemp seeds, for serving

Make the dressing: Whisk together the tahini, water, tamari, sesame oil, lime juice, garlic, maple syrup, and red pepper flakes until smooth. Set aside.

Cook the soba noodles according to package instructions, then drain and rinse under cold water to stop the cooking process. Return to the pan they were cooked in and toss with half of the prepared sesame sauce.

Divide the noodles among four resealable containers, then top with the edamame, carrots, cucumber, and tofu. Drizzle with the remaining sauce, the sesame seeds, and hemp seeds. Serve cold.

Lower FODMAP Options:

You can sub the tahini with peanut butter or almond butter.

Garlic is high in fructans. Replace with 1 teaspoon chives.

Supercharge It!

Bell pepper, broccoli, and sliced scallions would all taste great in this dish.

Make-Ahead Tips:

We love these glass containers for meal prep storage.

10 PLANT POINTS

Crispy Baked Tofu

This crispy baked tofu can be used anywhere throughout the meal plan: for extra protein, to top on salads, or to snack on its own. We'll use this recipe in our Sesame Noodle Prep Bowls in Week 3, and it can be substituted in for the peanut tofu in the Thai Bowls in Week 3 and added to the Nourishing Buddha Bowl in Week 4.

Serves 4

14 ounces firm or super-firm tofu
Olive oil cooking spray

Remove the tofu from the package and wrap it in a clean towel or paper towel. Place it on a plate, then put another plate on top of it. Place a few heavy items like cans or cookbooks on top of the tofu. Allow to sit for 30 minutes, or until most of the water has drained onto the towel.

Preheat the oven to 400°F.

Once the tofu is drained, place it on a cutting board and cut into desired shape. For Week 3 of the *Fiber Fueled* plan, rectangles and squares work well. Lightly spray a baking sheet with olive oil and place the tofu on it in a single layer, then spritz with more olive oil to ensure that tofu is well-coated.

Bake for 15 minutes. Remove from the oven and flip. Return to the oven and bake for 15 more minutes, or until the tofu is golden brown. Use in recipes throughout the week as needed. Store in a sealed container in the fridge.

1 PLANT POINT

Nourishing Buddha Bowl

This lunch bowl is our favorite "let's see what we can put together for a meal" recipe. It's a recipe but not really a recipe. It is inspired by a salad that I created at my fave restaurant in Charleston, Verde. But you can totally adapt it! The only must is the tahini dressing, which is so good, you'll want to put it on everything anyway.

We've included a loose list of things to add, but it's also customizable to whatever leftovers you have from the week. Think of this one as a clean-out-the-fridge type of meal.

Serves 1

Tahini Dressing

¼ cup tahini

2 tablespoons freshly squeezed lemon juice

1 garlic clove, minced

1 tablespoon olive oil

½ teaspoon salt

Bowl

½ cup chickpeas (or other cooked beans/lentil of choice)

2 to 3 cups salad greens

½ cup cooked grains

½ cup leftover Roasted Vegetables (recipe follows) or other chopped vegetables

Make the dressing: Whisk together the tahini, ⅓ cup water, the lemon juice, garlic, and olive oil. Season to taste with salt, as desired. Set aside.

Assemble: Place the chickpeas, salad greens, cooked grains, and other vegetables in a large bowl and drizzle with ¼ cup tahini dressing per bowl.

Low FODMAP Options:

Tahini is high in fructans. Reduce to 1 tablespoon, then increase the olive oil by 2 tablespoons and reduce the water by half.

Garlic is high FODMAP. Omit and use garlic-infused olive oil (see page 246) in place of the regular olive oil.

Chickpeas have moderate GOS. Limit to ¼ cup or use ½ cup canned lentils.

Millet, quinoa, brown rice, and white rice are low FODMAP grains.

Supercharge It!

When cooking your grains, add ½ teaspoon ground turmeric to your cooking water. Cook as directed.

6 PLANT POINTS

Roasted Vegetables

As mentioned, this bowl is a great way to use up leftover cooked grains and vegetables. If you don't have any, this is an easy go-to recipe.

Serves 2

1 cup chopped asparagus, woody ends removed
1 green bell pepper, chopped
1 cup broccoli florets, chopped
2 teaspoons olive oil
Pinch salt
Pinch freshly ground black pepper

Preheat the oven to 400°F.

Toss the asparagus, bell pepper, and broccoli with the olive oil, salt, and pepper until well coated. Place in a single layer on a rimmed baking sheet. Cook for 20 to 25 minutes, until tender.

Low FODMAP Options:

Asparagus is high FODMAP. Omit the asparagus and use zucchini or another low FODMAP vegetable.

DINNER

Thai Rainbow Bowls with Peanut Tofu

First off, the spicy peanut sauce makes my heart race a little. So. Good. We've added in higher FODMAP foods, like garlic, into this dish. If you notice symptoms coming back, make sure to check out the lower FODMAP options below.

Serves 2

½ cup uncooked brown rice

6 ounces firm or extra-firm tofu, drained, pressed, and cubed

Spicy Peanut Sauce

⅓ cup creamy peanut butter

1 tablespoon tamari

1 tablespoon 100% maple syrup

3 tablespoons freshly squeezed lime juice

¼ teaspoon crushed red pepper flakes, or more or less for spice preference

1 garlic clove, minced

2 tablespoons peanuts, finely chopped, plus more for garnish

3 tablespoons hot water

Salt and freshly ground black pepper

1 carrot, shaved into long, noodle-like strips with a vegetable peeler

1 cup sliced (half-moon shapes) cucumber

1 cup sliced Napa or red cabbage

½ red bell pepper, sliced

2 scallions (green parts only), chopped

Preheat the oven to 400°F.

Bring 1 cup of water to a boil in a medium saucepan over medium-high heat. Add the rice, cover, and reduce the heat to low. Simmer until the rice is tender, about 30 minutes then lightly fluff with a fork and set aside.

Place the tofu in a single layer on a rimmed nonstick baking sheet and cook for 25 minutes, or until lightly browned. If you aren't using a nonstick baking sheet, lightly spray with cooking spray. Remove the tofu from the oven, place in a shallow bowl, and set aside.

Make the sauce: Whisk together the peanut butter, tamari, maple syrup, lime juice, red pepper flakes, garlic, and peanuts until creamy and thick. Keep whisking, slowly whisking in hot water until the sauce is pourable. Season to taste with salt and pepper, then add 3 tablespoons of the sauce to the cooked tofu and toss to coat. Set aside.

Divide the cooked rice into two bowls and top with the tofu, carrots, cucumbers, cabbage, bell peppers, and scallions. Drizzle with the remaining Spicy Peanut Sauce and serve.

Make-Ahead Tips:

The tofu can be baked ahead of time and stored in an airtight container in the fridge. It won't be crispy after being stored in the fridge, so you can fry it in a lightly oiled skillet before serving, if desired.

The Spicy Peanut Sauce can be made ahead of time; store in an airtight container in the fridge for up to 4 days.

Low FODMAP Options:

Garlic is high in fructans. Omit and replace with 1 teaspoon sliced scallion greens.

Red, Savoy, and common cabbage are moderate FODMAP when you use more than ¾ cup per serving.

The white bulb of the scallion is high in fructans, so only use the green parts for low FODMAP.

Supercharge It!

Top with cilantro and/or hemp seeds.

10 PLANT POINTS

Lentil Bolognese with Spaghetti Squash

If you can't find spaghetti squash, no worries! Just substitute cooked pasta of choice. Boom. Ya good.

Serves 2

1 large spaghetti squash, halved and seeds scooped out

1 tablespoon plus 1 teaspoon olive oil

¾ teaspoon salt, plus more to taste

¼ teaspoon freshly ground black pepper, plus more to taste

1 medium shallot, minced

4 garlic cloves, minced

2 medium carrots, chopped

2 celery stalks, chopped

4 cups tomato sauce

¾ cup dry red lentils

1 teaspoon dried basil

1 teaspoon dried oregano

1 pinch crushed red pepper flakes

Pepita Parmesan (recipe follows), for serving

Preheat the oven to 400°F.

Rub the squash with 1 teaspoon olive oil and season with ¼ teaspoon salt and ¼ teaspoon pepper. Place the squash cut-side down on a rimmed baking sheet and roast for 45 to 50 minutes, until tender. Remove and let cool until able to touch, then use a fork to scrape out the spaghetti-like strands. Set aside.

Make the sauce: Heat the remaining 1 tablespoon of olive oil in a large rimmed skillet over medium heat and add the shallot and garlic.

Sauté, stirring frequently, for about 3 minutes, until soft and fragrant, taking care not to burn.

Add the carrots and celery and cook for 4 to 5 minutes, until the vegetables are softened. Add the tomato sauce, lentils, basil, oregano, red pepper flakes, and ½ cup water. Raise the heat to bring the mixture to a low boil, then reduce the heat to low. Cover and cook for about 20 minutes, stirring occasionally, until the lentils are tender. If the mixture is cooking too quickly, add more water to prevent it from drying out. Add in the remaining ½ teaspoon of salt. Add more salt and pepper to taste.

Divide the spaghetti squash strands between two bowls and top with the lentil Bolognese and additional garnishes, if using.

Low FODMAP Option:

Shallots are high in fructans. Omit and use shallot-infused olive oil (either use store-bought Fody brand or make your own) in place of the regular olive oil, or sub in ¼ cup scallion greens.

Garlic is high in FODMAP and fructans. Omit and use ½ cup chives, or sub garlic-infused olive oil (see page 246) in place of the plain olive oil.

Celery is high FODMAP. Reduce to ⅔ medium celery stalk.

Tomato sauce may contain onion and garlic. Look for brands that contain just tomato. If substituting with marinara sauce, then look for these low FODMAP options if you are sensitive to fructans. We like Fody Tomato Basil Pasta Sauce, Fody Marinara Pasta Sauce, and Rao's Homemade Sensitive Marinara Sauce.

Dry red lentils have moderate GOS. Sub 1 cup canned lentils.

Supercharge It!

Top with the Pepita Parmesan, chopped fresh basil, and chopped fresh parsley.

7 PLANT POINTS

Pepita Parmesan

½ cup slivered almonds (20 whole almonds)

¼ cup raw pepitas

3 tablespoons nutritional yeast

1 teaspoon salt

Place the almonds, pepitas, nutritional yeast, and salt in the base of a food processor and process until a fine powder forms, taking care not to turn it into almond butter. Store in the fridge for up to 2 weeks or in the freezer for up to 6 months.

Low FODMAP Option:

Slivered almonds are high in GOS. Decrease the quantity to 10 nuts.

Buffalo Chickpea Salad

We simply had to have this flavor in the four-week plan. Spicy buffalo chickpeas mix with sweet hummus dressing. A match made in heaven!

Makes 2 salads

Sweet Hummus Dressing

¼ cup Pumpkin Hummus (page 276) or other hummus

2 teaspoons 100% maple syrup

2 tablespoons red wine vinegar or freshly squeezed lemon juice

2 teaspoons hot water

Buffalo Chickpeas

½ cup canned chickpeas, drained and rinsed

2 teaspoons garlic-infused olive oil (see page 246)

1 tablespoon hot sauce, like Texas Pete

¼ teaspoon minced garlic

Pinch salt

Salad

4 cups chopped romaine lettuce

¼ avocado, sliced

¼ cup halved cherry tomatoes

Make the dressing: Whisk together the hummus, maple syrup, and vinegar until creamy and smooth. Keep whisking while slowly adding in the hot water. The dressing should be thick but pourable. Add more water as needed.

Make the chickpeas: Toss the chickpeas with the infused olive oil, hot sauce, garlic, and salt. Heat a skillet over medium heat. Add the chickpeas and sauté for 3 minutes, or until the chickpeas start to dry out and are heated through. Use the back of a spoon to gently mash some of the chickpeas together, keeping most of them whole. Remove from the heat and set aside.

Make the salad: Toss the romaine with the dressing, then gently toss in the avocado, tomatoes, and buffalo chickpeas. Divide between two bowls and serve immediately.

Low FODMAP Options:

Use the FODMAP-friendly Pumpkin Hummus (page 276) in this recipe as most prepared hummus will contain garlic and/or onion. Limit chickpeas to a single ¼ cup serving per person. Garlic is high in fructans. Substitute 1 teaspoon chives.

Make-Ahead Option:

Prepare the Sweet Hummus Dressing and Buffalo Chickpeas ahead of time. Before serving, warm the chickpeas, then assemble as directed.

7 PLANT POINTS

Gumbo

While this recipe comes together easily, it does take time for the vegetables to cook down and the gumbo to simmer. If that's too much on a weeknight, then add this recipe to your prep list for Sunday and plan on cooking just the rice that night. Freeze half for use in Week 4 and place the remaining half in the fridge until ready to eat.

Serves 4

Salt and freshly ground black pepper
2 cups uncooked brown rice
3 tablespoons olive oil
1 medium onion, diced
1 green bell pepper, diced
3 celery stalks, diced
3 garlic cloves, minced
Salt
¼ cup all-purpose flour
2 teaspoons smoked paprika
2 teaspoons dried thyme
1 teaspoon freshly ground black pepper
1 teaspoon dried oregano
4 cups vegetable broth or Biome Broth (page 249)
One 14-ounce can fire-roasted tomatoes, drained
One 14-ounce can kidney beans, drained and rinsed
1½ cups frozen, sliced okra
2 tablespoons vegan Worcestershire sauce

Make the rice: Bring 4 cups water and a pinch salt to a boil in a large pot over medium-high heat, then add the rice. Reduce the heat to low, cover, and let the rice cook for about 45 minutes, until tender.

Make the gumbo: Heat the olive oil in a large stockpot over medium heat. Add the onion, bell pepper, celery, and garlic along with a pinch of salt and cook, stirring occasionally, for about 15 minutes, until the vegetables are lightly browned and cooked through.

Sprinkle the flour on the vegetables and stir, cooking for 2 to 3 more minutes, until the flour is slightly toasted and smells nutty. Add in the paprika, thyme, black pepper, and oregano and stir together, cooking another 30 to 60 seconds, until just fragrant.

Add in the broth, tomatoes, beans, okra, and Worcestershire sauce and whisk together to combine, trying to scrape up any browned bits of vegetable and flour on the bottom of the pan. Raise the heat to medium-high and bring to a boil. Once boiling, reduce the heat and simmer, stirring occasionally, until thick, about 30 minutes.

Divide 1 cup of the cooked rice between two bowls and top with Gumbo. Reserve the remaining rice for Kimchi Fried Rice (page 305) and freeze the remaining Gumbo for dinner next week.

Low FODMAP Options:
Onion is high in fructans and has moderate GOS. Omit and sub ½ cup scallion greens.

A quarter of a green bell pepper contains moderate FODMAPs. Reduce the amount used in the recipe to ½ green bell pepper, or use a whole red bell pepper instead of a green bell pepper.

Three celery stalks have moderate mannitol. Reduce to 1 celery stalk.

Garlic is high in fructans. Omit and sub garlic-infused olive oil (see page 246) for the regular olive oil.

Wheat flour is high in GOS and fructans. Sub gluten-free flour.

Kidney beans are high in GOS and fructans. Sub 1 cup chickpeas or canned lentils.

Meal Prep Tip:

Both the rice and the gumbo make an appearance later in the plan. Save 2 cups cooked rice for Kimchi Fried Rice (below) and freeze the remaining Gumbo for dinner in Week 4.

If making this on Week 3, then make the full 1¼ cups of brown rice to use leftovers for Kimchi Fried Rice (below). If just making the gumbo, then cook ½ cup of dry brown rice.

Supercharge It!

Top with chopped parsley.

7 PLANT POINTS

Kimchi Fried Rice

This fried rice gets a *Fiber Fueled* boost from the addition of kimchi, a Korean staple of fermented cabbage and vegetables. Alex really likes Sunja's Kimchi; use it if you can find it.

Serves 2

One 16-ounce jar kimchi

2 teaspoons toasted sesame oil, plus more if needed

3 scallions, sliced

8 ounces firm tofu, drained and pressed

3 garlic cloves, minced

1 tablespoon fresh grated ginger

2 bunches baby bok choy, thinly sliced

4 ounces shiitake mushrooms, thinly sliced

1 tablespoon tamari, plus more if needed

2 cups cooked and cooled brown rice, reserved from Gumbo recipe (page 303)

2 teaspoons rice wine vinegar

Drain the kimchi in a colander, reserving the liquid. Roughly chop the kimchi a few times into bite-size pieces, then set aside.

Heat the sesame oil in a large skillet over medium-high heat. Add the scallions and cook, stirring frequently, for 2 to 3 minutes, until tender. Crumble in the tofu and stir to combine. Cook for an additional 2 to 3 minutes, until lightly browned. Stir in the garlic and ginger.

Add in the bok choy and mushrooms and cook for another 2 to 3 minutes, until the bok choy is bright green and tender.

Add in the kimchi and tamari and cook until just heated through.

Add in the rice, 1 tablespoon reserved kimchi brine, and the vinegar and cook, stirring frequently, for 3 to 4 minutes, until the mixture is heated through. Season to taste, adding more tamari, toasted sesame oil, or kimchi brine, as desired. Serve immediately.

Low FODMAP Options:
Kimchi is high in fructans. Many kimchi brands contain garlic, so if you are sensitive to fructans, then you can either omit the kimchi altogether or select a different recipe for dinner tonight.
Use only the green parts of scallions for low FODMAP.
Garlic is high FODMAP and fructan. Omit and use 2 teaspoons garlic-infused olive oil (see page 246) instead.
A 1-cup serving of bok choy is FODMAP friendly. Over 1⅓ cups per serving is moderate in sorbitol.
Shiitake mushrooms are high in mannitol. Substitute oyster mushrooms or omit.

Supercharge It!
Top with sliced nori strips, sesame seeds, sliced scallions, or pickled ginger.

7 PLANT POINTS

Lentil Masala

It's no secret that we are big fans of Indian food. Packed with fragrant, antioxidant-rich spices, aromatics, vegetables, and pulses, Indian cuisine is a great way to enjoy traditional *Fiber Fueled* cuisine. This simplified lentil masala uses cashew cream, a delicious, dairy-free alternative that tastes just as rich and luscious. If you haven't made cashew cream before, this is one recipe that you'll likely turn to over and over again; it works great in any recipe that calls for heavy cream.

Serves 2

Cilantro-Lime Rice

½ cup uncooked basmati or brown rice

Salt

2 tablespoons freshly squeezed lime juice

¼ cup finely chopped cilantro

Lentils

2 teaspoons olive oil or Biome Broth (page 249)

½ yellow or white onion, chopped

1 inch fresh ginger, grated or minced

2 garlic cloves, minced

Pinch salt and freshly ground black pepper

½ teaspoon garam masala

½ teaspoon chili powder

⅛ teaspoon ground cinnamon

2 tablespoons tomato paste

½ cup dried green or brown lentils

Cashew Cream

¼ cup raw cashews (20 whole cashews)

⅓ cup warm water

Freshly squeezed lime juice, for serving

Fresh cilantro, for serving

Make the rice: In a small saucepan, bring 1 cup of cold water to a boil over medium-high heat. Add the rice, reduce the heat to low, cover, and cook according to the package instructions, until the rice is tender. Stir in ¼ teaspoon salt, 1 tablespoon of the lime juice, and the cilantro. Set aside.

Make the lentils: Heat the olive oil in a large skillet over medium heat. Add in the onion, ginger, and garlic and cook for 5 to 7 minutes, until softened. Add the salt and pepper along with the garam masala, chili powder, and cinnamon. Cook for 1 minute, until fragrant.

Add the tomato paste and cook for 1 more minute, until dark red and fragrant. Add the lentils and 2 cups cold water, then bring to a boil. Reduce the heat to medium-low, cover, and cook for 30 minutes, stirring occasionally, until the lentils are tender and most of the water has been absorbed.

Make the cashew cream: Combine the cashews and warm water in a blender and blend until very creamy and thick. Depending on the power of your blender, this may take up to 5 minutes.

Stir the cashew cream and remaining 1 tablespoon lime juice into the lentils and season to taste, adding more salt as needed. Serve over the reserved cilantro-lime rice, topping with more cilantro and lime juice as desired.

Low FODMAP Option:

Yellow or white onions have moderate GOS and are high in fructans. Omit and substitute with ¼ cup scallion greens.

Garlic is high in fructans. Omit and use 2 teaspoons garlic-infused olive oil (see page 246) in place of the regular olive oil.

Some garam masala contains garlic and onion, so make sure to check the ingredient list.

Lentils have moderate GOS. Reduce to ¼ cup dry green or brown lentils and reduce the water by half.

20 cashews is high FODMAP. Omit the cashew cream for a less creamy version of the Lentil Masala.

6 PLANT POINTS

SNACKS, DRINKS, AND DESSERTS

The Green Drink

This tart drink is a mix between a fruit smoothie and a limeade! Very refreshing, it's a great midafternoon pick-me-up. For a heartier snack, pair with Turmeric Energy Bites (page 310) or Chickpea Cookie Dough Bites (page 279).

Serves 2
2 cups chopped honeydew melon*
4 kiwis, peeled
Zest and juice of 1 lime
10 mint leaves
2 cups crushed ice

Place the honeydew, kiwi, lime zest, lime juice, mint, ice, and ½ cup water into a blender and process until smooth. Divide between two glasses and serve.

Low FODMAP Options:
Reduce melon to 1 cup total for the recipe, or use 1½ cups cantaloupe for the entire recipe.

4 PLANT POINTS

Speedy Edamame

We call this Speedy Edamame because it comes together in just
5 minutes and is the perfect plant-powered snack. Enjoy with salt,
or a pinch of chili powder or red pepper flakes if you like things spicy.

Serves 2
½ teaspoon salt
1 cup frozen or fresh edamame in pods
Coarse finishing salt

Place 3 cups water and the salt in a medium saucepan and bring to a
boil over high heat. Add the edamame and cook for about 5 minutes,
until the edamame are tender and easily release from their pod.
Drain and toss with a pinch of coarse finishing salt, like kosher salt
or fleur de sel. Serve warm or cold.

Make-Ahead Tip:
The edamame can be made ahead of time and enjoyed cold or reheated in the
microwave right before eating.

1 PLANT POINT

Turmeric Energy Bites

Turmeric contains the plant compound curcumin, which is known for
its anti-inflammatory and antioxidant properties. It is also what gives
curry its vibrant yellow color. We added it to these bites with a touch of
lemon for a sweet ball that's perfect for a snack between meals or a
sweet after-dinner treat. Once it hits your lips . . . it's so good!

Makes 16 to 18 bites
1⅓ cups rolled oats
¼ cup chopped or sliced almonds

¼ cup hemp seeds

½ cup almond or peanut butter

¼ cup 100% maple syrup

1 teaspoon lemon zest

2 tablespoons freshly squeezed lemon juice

1 teaspoon ground turmeric

Pinch salt

Pinch freshly ground black pepper

Add the oats, almonds, and hemp seeds to a medium bowl. Mix in the almond butter, maple syrup, lemon zest, lemon juice, turmeric, salt, and pepper until well combined.

Cover a small tray or plate with parchment paper. Roll the mixture into tablespoon-size balls and place on a parchment paper–lined tray.

Place the tray in the refrigerator to chill until set, then transfer to an airtight container and keep in the fridge for up to 1 week or the freezer for up to 2 months.

Low FODMAP Option:

Almonds are higher in FODMAPs (GOS) but a serving size of 10 nuts or 1 tablespoon of almond butter are okay if you're sensitive. One and a half tablespoons of almond butter has moderate GOS. Please pay attention to how you feel when increasing certain foods higher in FODMAPs this week and make adjustments to the recipes with the lower FODMAP options as necessary.

Peanut butter is lower in FODMAPs than almond butter.

Supercharge It!

Add 1 tablespoon flaxseeds or chia seeds (or both!) to get more omega-3 fatty acids and fiber.

4 PLANT POINTS

Chocolate Banana Nice Cream

You scream, I scream, we all scream for nice cream! This chocolate banana nice cream is the perfect after-dinner dessert.

Note: To make a cherry version, remove the chocolate and add in ⅓ cup frozen pitted cherries instead.

Serves 2
4 peeled, frozen, chopped bananas
1 to 2 teaspoons cocoa powder
½ teaspoon vanilla extract

Add the bananas, cocoa powder, and vanilla to the base of a food processor and blend until very creamy and the consistency of soft serve.

Note: Leftovers don't keep well, so halve the recipe if you don't plan on eating the entire recipe in one sitting.

Low FODMAP Options:
If you're using cherries instead of cocoa powder, reduce the serving to 2 cherries if you are sensitive to fructose.
1 medium unripe banana is considered low FODMAP. Ripe bananas (slightly brown) are higher in fructose. One-third of a ripe banana has the green light, and ½ of a ripe banana has moderate fructans.

2 PLANT POINTS

Mushroom Hot Cocoa

Keep calm and mushroom on. We know that mushrooms in cocoa sounds a little odd, but these aren't your traditional mushrooms! We like a single powder or a blend of powdered Reishi, Lion's Mane, and/or Cordyceps as these medicinal mushrooms are adaptogens and have been shown to help with stress, energy levels, and more restful sleep.

Adding the peanut or almond butter helps to make this hot cocoa very rich, and the added fat helps with satiety.

Pro Tip: Medicinal Mushrooms
For the mushroom hot cocoa, choose the mushroom that fits your goals: Immune boosting—Reishi; Focus—Lion's Mane; Energy—Cordyceps.

Serves 2

2 teaspoons mushroom powder

1 tablespoon 100% maple syrup

1 tablespoon peanut butter or almond butter

2 tablespoons unsweetened cocoa powder

Pinch salt

½ teaspoon ground cinnamon

2½ cups dairy-free milk

Add the mushroom powder, maple syrup, peanut butter, cocoa powder, salt, cinnamon, and milk to a blender and puree until creamy.

Place the blended cocoa mixture into a small saucepan and warm over medium heat, whisking vigorously right before serving until frothy and well blended.

Taste and adjust the flavor as needed. Divide into two mugs and serve warm.

3 PLANT POINTS

Week 4

You should feel proud of how far you've come. This is the fourth week! You are almost ready to transition into the FF365 program. Make sure to keep track of your favorite recipes and any food sensitivities that you see coming up. Post your results to #fiberfueled4weeks. Let's embolden and support others to take on the same quest that you have—to improve your health through diet and lifestyle.

WEEK 4 SHOPPING LIST

Produce

- ☐ 1 medium piece fresh ginger
- ☐ 4 large lemons
- ☐ 3 large green bell peppers
- ☐ 2 yellow bell peppers
- ☐ 1 large orange bell pepper
- ☐ 1 ounce dried shiitake mushrooms
- ☐ 3 medium yellow or white onions
- ☐ 1 red onion
- ☐ 1 pound carrots
- ☐ 1 pound celery hearts
- ☐ 1 large cucumber
- ☐ 1 large mango
- ☐ 1 small jicama
- ☐ 2 pints cherry tomatoes
- ☐ One 10-ounce bag spinach leaves
- ☐ 6 bananas
- ☐ 2 kiwis
- ☐ One 5-ounce package leafy salad greens
- ☐ One 100-gram container broccoli sprouts
- ☐ 4 large avocados
- ☐ 1 bunch fresh chives

- ☐ 2 bunches kale (lactino or curly)
- ☐ 2 jalapeños
- ☐ 2 bunches fresh cilantro
- ☐ 1 bunch fresh basil
- ☐ 1 pint strawberries
- ☐ 1 pint berries of choice
- ☐ One 8-ounce bag dates
- ☐ One 10-ounce package walnuts
- ☐ One 5-ounce package cashews
- ☐ One 8-ounce package almonds
- ☐ 5 limes
- ☐ 1 head garlic
- ☐ 2 large oranges
- ☐ 1 large grapefruit
- ☐ 2 bunches scallions
- ☐ 1 head broccoli
- ☐ 1 large tomato
- ☐ One 5-ounce bag arugula
- ☐ One 64-ounce container almond milk
- ☐ One 2-ounce jar sesame seeds
- ☐ One 15-ounce can or container low-sodium vegetable broth
- ☐ 8 ounces baked tofu
- ☐ 1 package chai tea (in bags)
- ☐ One 8-ounce package tempeh
- ☐ One 1-ounce bag wakame
- ☐ One 16-ounce bag brown lentils
- ☐ Four 15-ounce cans chickpeas
- ☐ One 15-ounce can white beans
- ☐ One 15-ounce can coconut milk
- ☐ One 15-ounce container Sriracha
- ☐ One 15-ounce container bread crumbs
- ☐ One 15-ounce can tomato sauce

☐ Three 15-ounce cans diced tomatoes

☐ Two 15-ounce cans black beans

☐ One 15-ounce can kidney beans

☐ One 15-ounce can pinto beans

☐ Two 15-ounce cans cannellini beans

Jarred marinara sauce (Rao's and Fody are low FODMAP; see Chickpea Meatballs [page 329] for more details)

1 package sub rolls

1 package whole-grain buns

2 ounces soba noodles

One 8-ounce bag elbow noodles

One 8-ounce bag dried pasta of choice

One 8-ounce bag whole-grain spaghetti

One 14-ounce bag white rice

Bay leaves

Garlic powder

Dry mustard

1-ounce package nori sheets

1 loaf sourdough bread

1 16-ounce package firm tofu, packed in water

Week 4—Drinks, Snacks, and Dessert

Remember, these recipes are to be enjoyed whenever the moment feels right.

Drink Recipe: Turmeric Latte (page 340)

Snack Recipe #1: White Bean Hummus with vegetables (page 341)

Snack Recipe #2: Omega-3 Balls (page 342)

Dessert Recipe #1: Strawberry Cheesecake Bites (page 343)

Dessert Recipe #2: Snicker Bites (page 345)

Week 4—Quick-Fix Menu

Friendly Note: Now that we're four weeks into the plan, it's okay to increase the amount of berries you eat.

Quick-Fix Breakfast: Superfood Smoothie Bowl (page 225)

Quick-Fix Lunch: Chickpea Meatball Sandwich (page 329)

Quick-Fix Dinner: Leftover 4-Bean Chili (page 326) with White
 Bean Hummus (page 341) on sourdough

Quick-Fix Snack: Handful of almonds

Quick-Fix Dessert: Bowl of berries

Week 4 Meal Prep

Week 4 Recommended Prep

White Bean Hummus (page 341)

Nourishing Buddha Bowl (page 295)

Omega-3 Balls (page 342)

Week 4 Optional Prep

Chickpea Meatballs (page 329) for dinner on Day 3 and lunch again on Day 4. Extra meatballs can be used for quick-fix lunch anytime this week.

4-Bean Chili (page 326)

Cook the lentils ahead of time for Lentil Sloppy Joes (page 332) for
 dinner on Day 5

Banana Baked Oatmeal (page 320)

DAY 1 (USUALLY SUNDAY)

Meal	Recipe	Page	Plant Points
Breakfast	Gluten-Free Pancakes	262	2
Lunch	Supercharged Miso Soup	322	8
Dinner	4-Bean Chili	326	7–10

DAY 2

Meal	Recipe	Page	Plant Points
Breakfast	Superfood Smoothie Bowl with Crispy Oat Granola	Smoothie Bowl: 225 Crispy Oat Granola: 228	12
Lunch	Nourishing Buddha Bowl with Tahini Dressing	295	6
Dinner	Nothing Fishy Sushi Wraps	324	6

DAY 3

Meal	Recipe	Page	Plant Points
Breakfast	Banana Baked Oatmeal	320	4
Lunch	Nothing Fishy Sushi Bowl	Nothing Fishy Sushi Wraps: 324	6
Dinner	Chickpea Meatballs Pasta Marinara and Quick Garlic Broccoli	Chickpea Meatballs: 329 Quick Garlic Broccoli: 331	5

DAY 4

Meal	Recipe	Page	Plant Points
Breakfast	Creamy Chai Oats	321	5
Lunch	Chickpea Meatballs on sourdough sub roll	Chickpea Meatballs: 329	4
Dinner	Leftover Gumbo with brown rice	Gumbo: 303	8

DAY 5

Meal	Recipe	Page	Plant Points
Breakfast	Banana Baked Oatmeal	320	4
Lunch	Leftover 4-Bean Chili or Chili Mac	4-Bean Chili: 326 Chili Mac: 327	7+
Dinner	Lentil Sloppy Joes with Jicama Fries	Lentil Sloppy Joes: 332 Jicama Fries: 333	7

DAY 6

Meal	Recipe	Page	Plant Points
Breakfast	Chocolate Peanut Butter Super Smoothie	287	4+
Lunch	Chickpea and Avocado Sandwich with Citrus and Mint Salad	Chickpea and Avocado Sandwich: 334 Citrus and Mint Salad: 265	7+
Dinner	Tuscan Kale Soup with Down 'n' Dirty Kale Salad	Tuscan Kale Soup: 335 Down 'n' Dirty Kale Salad: 233	13–16

DAY 7

Meal	Recipe	Page	Plant Points
Breakfast	Spicy Breakfast Tacos	288	6
Lunch	Leftover Tuscan Kale Soup with sourdough bread and White Bean Hummus	Tuscan Kale Soup: 335 White Bean Hummus: 341	14–16
Dinner	Sunday Pasta	337	6+

BREAKFAST

Banana Baked Oatmeal

Baked oatmeal is one of our favorite warm breakfasts. While this one is delicious right out of the pan, we recommend enjoying it warm, topped with cold almond milk, chopped nuts, and extra berries.

To prepare ahead, assemble everything the night before to bake in the morning or prep on Sunday and reheat with a little more almond milk as it will dry out slightly in the fridge.

Serves 4, with leftovers for later in the week

1 large banana, sliced

1½ cups quick-cooking oats

2 tablespoons ground flaxseeds

½ teaspoon ground cinnamon

1 teaspoon baking powder

¼ teaspoon salt

¾ cup almond milk or other dairy-free milk

⅓ cup 100% maple syrup

2 tablespoons organic sunflower oil

1 teaspoon vanilla extract

¼ cup chopped walnuts or other chopped nut

Preheat the oven to 350°F. Lightly spray an 8 x 8-inch baking dish.

Place the sliced bananas in a single row on the bottom of the pan and set aside.

In a medium bowl, whisk together the oats, flaxseeds, cinnamon, baking powder, and salt.

In a separate medium bowl, whisk together the almond milk, maple syrup, sunflower oil, and vanilla. Add to the oat mixture and stir together until combined. Stir in the chopped nuts and gently top the sliced bananas in the baking dish with the oatmeal. Place in the oven and bake for 30 minutes, or until golden brown and set.

Low FODMAP Options:
Quick-cooking oats have moderate GOS and fructans. Sub rolled oats.

Supercharge It!
Top with berries, almond milk, and chopped nuts.

4 PLANT POINTS

Creamy Chai Oats

All the flavors of spicy, comforting chai in your morning bowl of creamy oats.

Makes 2 servings
1 chai tea bag
1½ cups unsweetened almond milk
½ teaspoon ground cinnamon
¼ teaspoon ground cardamom
¼ teaspoon ground nutmeg
1 cup old-fashioned oats
1 teaspoon ground flaxseeds
1 teaspoon chia seeds
1 tablespoon hemp seeds
1 banana, mashed
1 teaspoon vanilla extract
Pinch salt
1 teaspoon 100% maple syrup (optional)

In a medium saucepan, bring the chai tea bag, ½ cup water, almond milk, cinnamon, cardamom, and nutmeg to a boil over medium heat.

Reduce the heat to low and simmer for 2 minutes, stirring occasionally.

Remove the tea bag and bring to a boil over medium-high heat. Stir in the oats, flax, chia, and hemp seeds. Reduce the heat to medium-low and cook for about 3 minutes, until the oats are thick.

Stir in the mashed banana and cook for 1 more minute. Remove from the heat, stir in the vanilla and salt, then cover and allow to finish cooking for 5 minutes. Stir in the maple syrup, if using, and serve.

Low FODMAP Options:

A ripe banana is high in fructose, but a greener banana will be lower FODMAP.

Supercharge It!

Top this oatmeal with your favorite berries for extra sweetness and Plant Points.

Make-Ahead Tips:

You can make this ahead of time and store in an airtight container in the fridge. Enjoy warm or cold.

5 PLANT POINTS

LUNCH

Supercharged Miso Soup

Miso is a paste made from fermented soybeans and very common in Asian cuisine. This soup is warm, comforting, and delicious.

Serves 2

2 ounces soba noodles

2 cups Biome Broth (page 249)

1 tablespoon wakame seaweed

¼ cup white miso paste

½ cup chopped baby spinach

½ cup chopped scallions

¼ cup firm tofu, drained and cubed

¼ cup rehydrated shiitake mushrooms

Bring a medium pot of water to a boil over medium-high heat. Cook the soba noodles according to the package instructions, then drain and rinse with cool water to stop the cooking. Set aside.

In the same pot, bring 2 cups of cold water and the broth to a boil over medium-high heat. Add the wakame, reduce the heat, and simmer over low heat for about 5 minutes.

In a small bowl, combine the miso with 1 to 2 teaspoons warm water to thin it out to the consistency of a thick, creamy sauce. Set aside.

Add the baby spinach, scallions, tofu, and shiitake mushrooms to the broth. Bring to a boil over medium-high heat, then cover, reduce the heat to low, and simmer for 5 minutes.

Remove from the heat and stir in the miso paste and cooked soba noodles. Serve.

Low FODMAP Options:

The white parts of scallions are high in fructans. Use only the green parts.

Supercharge Options:

Top with sesame seeds and/or sliced scallions for an added texture bonus and flavor boost.

8 PLANT POINTS

Nothing Fishy Sushi Wraps

Nothing fishy here! This might be one of our favorite recipes in the entire book. Be warned, the sriracha mayo is addictive; enjoy it here, on sandwiches, and anywhere else you want a spicy hit of creamy flavor.

We call these wraps, but they are assembled like a lettuce wrap. Pile everything high onto toasted nori sheets, loosely wrap, and enjoy. We like to serve these disassembled, with bowls of all the toppings for everyone to top and eat as they choose.

This recipe makes enough for leftovers as Nothing Fishy Sushi Bowls. They are exactly like they sound: Toss everything in a bowl, cover with leftover sriracha mayo, and enjoy.

Serves 4, with leftovers for Nothing Fishy Sushi Bowls
Sriracha Mayo
½ cup raw cashews, soaked in 1 cup boiling water for 10 minutes and drained
1 tablespoon freshly squeezed lime juice
1 tablespoon sriracha
2 teaspoons 100% maple syrup
2 teaspoons tamari
½ teaspoon salt

1½ cups white rice (short-grain rice will stick together more easily, but any rice will work)
2 teaspoons tamari
6 toasted nori sheets, cut into quarters
1 cucumber, peeled and sliced into strips
1 large ripe mango, peeled and sliced into strips
8 ounces baked tofu, teriyaki flavor, sliced

1 large avocado, pitted and sliced thin

Sesame seeds, for topping

Make the mayo: Add the cashews to the base of a blender with ¼ cup cold water, the lime juice, sriracha, maple syrup, tamari, and salt. Blend until very creamy and smooth, scraping down the sides as needed.

Assemble the wraps: Bring 3 cups of water to a boil over medium-high heat in a large pot and add the rice. Reduce the heat to low, cover, and cook for 15 to 20 minutes, until the rice is tender (you might have to add a few minutes of cook time if you're using brown rice). Toss the warm rice with the vinegar and tamari. If you are using leftover cooked rice, add in a little warm water so the rice sticks together easily.

Press together a small handful of warm rice to make a ball, then press on top of a quartered sheet of toasted nori. Top with the cucumber, mango, tofu, and avocado.

Drizzle with the mayo and sprinkle with sesame seeds. Fold the wraps together and enjoy, dipping into more spicy mayo as desired!

To make bowls, toss all the remaining ingredients together.

Low FODMAP Options:

Cashews are high in GOS and have moderate fructans. The amount of cashews used in this recipe may still be low enough for you to tolerate if you are sensitive to GOS or fructans.

A quarter cup mango has moderate fructose; ½ cup has high fructose. If sensitive to fructose, reduce the amount so that only 3 tablespoons are portioned into 1 serving (¾ cup total).

Half an avocado is high in sorbitol. If sensitive to sorbitol, reduce so that only ⅛ avocado is portioned into 1 serving.

Make Ahead Tips:
For the Nothing Fishy Sushi Bowls, pack rice, toppings, and leftover sriracha mayo separately into airtight containers in the fridge. When ready to assemble, toss everything together and enjoy.

6 PLANT POINTS

DINNER

4-Bean Chili

You'll enjoy this 4-bean chili for dinner one night, then as Chili Mac later in the week. For a heartier meal, serve over cooked grains of choice, like quinoa. This recipe contains many high FODMAP ingredients, so sub Butternut Squash and Quinoa Chili (page 266) if necessary.

Makes 6 servings
1 tablespoon olive oil
1 white or yellow onion, chopped
1 yellow bell pepper, chopped
2 garlic cloves, minced
3 tablespoons chili powder, plus more to taste
1 tablespoon ground cumin, plus more to taste
2 teaspoons dried oregano, plus more to taste
2 cups low-sodium vegetable broth
1 cup tomato sauce
One 15-ounce can diced tomatoes
One 15-ounce can black beans
One 15-ounce can kidney beans
One 15-ounce can pinto beans

One 15-ounce can cannellini beans

¼ teaspoon salt, plus more to taste

Heat the olive oil in a large saucepan over medium heat until shimmering. Add the onion, bell pepper, and garlic and cook for 8 to 10 minutes, stirring occasionally, until the onion is translucent. Add the chili powder, cumin, and oregano and cook for 30 to 60 seconds, until fragrant.

Add the broth, tomato sauce, tomatoes, black beans, kidney beans, pinto beans, cannellini beans, and salt and raise the heat to medium-high to bring to a boil. Reduce the heat to low and simmer uncovered for 30 to 45 minutes, stirring occasionally, until the mixture is thick and the flavors have developed. Season to taste, as desired.

Serve, reserving 3 cups of the chili to make Chili Mac (see below).

Chili Mac

Easy Cheese Sauce

¼ cup cashews, soaked in boiling water for 30 minutes, then drained

½ orange bell pepper, roughly chopped

½ cup unsweetened almond milk

1 heaping tablespoon nutritional yeast, plus more to taste

1 teaspoon chili powder, plus more to taste

¼ teaspoon salt, plus more to taste

Chili Mac

2 cups cooked elbow noodles

3 cups reserved 4-Bean Chili

Place the cashews, bell pepper, almond milk, nutritional yeast, chili powder, and salt in the base of a food processor and puree until very creamy and smooth. Season to taste, adding in more salt, chili powder, or nutritional yeast as desired.

Cook the noodles according to the package instructions until al dente, then drain and set aside.

Warm the reserved chili, then add in the cooked noodles and cheese sauce. Stir together and enjoy!

Low FODMAP Options:

Tomato sauce may contain onion and garlic. If you are sensitive to fructans, look for these low FODMAP tomato sauce options: We like Fody Tomato Basil Pasta Sauce, Fody Marinara Pasta Sauce, and Rao's Homemade Sensitive Marinara Sauce.

Cashews are high in GOS and have moderate fructans. You can sub the ¼ cup cashews with ½ cup walnuts. Soak the walnuts overnight before using, then make according to the recipe above.

If you're sensitive to fructans in the wheat in the elbow noodles, sub quinoa or rice-based pasta.

Black beans are high in GOS and have moderate fructans.

Kidney beans are high in GOS and fructans.

Pinto beans are high in GOS and fructans.

Cannellini beans are high FODMAP.

Meal Prep Tip:

Make this chili on Sunday to enjoy for dinner on Sunday and lunch on Thursday, with the option for Chili Mac instead of chili that day.

Supercharge It!

Top with sliced scallions, chopped cilantro, and sliced jalapeños.

7+ PLANT POINTS

Chickpea Meatballs

You'll meal-prep these meatballs to be used with pasta, marinara sauce, and quick garlic broccoli for dinner one night, then tucked into a sub roll with the remaining pasta sauce for lunch the next day.

Any leftovers can be individually frozen, then stored in the freezer. Note that these will hold their shape when warmed through but may start to crumble if placed in sauce for a long period of time.

Makes 18 meatballs

1½ tablespoons ground flaxseed

3 cups canned chickpeas, drained and rinsed (½ cup serving is yellow light, GOS)

¾ cup walnuts

¾ cup bread crumbs, plus more as needed

3 tablespoons olive oil, plus more for drizzling

1½ teaspoons dried oregano

1½ teaspoons dried basil

1½ teaspoons dried parsley

¾ teaspoon salt

Freshly ground black pepper

Pasta Marinara

6 to 8 ounces dried pasta of your choice

2 cups marinara sauce

6 Chickpea Meatballs

Pepita Parmesan (page 301; optional)

Sandwich

1 cup marinara sauce

6 Chickpea Meatballs

2 sub rolls

Preheat the oven to 450°F. Lightly oil a rimmed baking sheet or line with parchment paper and set aside.

Mix together ¼ cup water and the ground flaxseeds in a bowl and set aside to gel. Place the chickpeas and walnuts in the base of a food processor and pulse until very finely chopped.

Remove the chickpea mixture from the food processor and place in a large bowl. Add the flaxseed mixture, bread crumbs, olive oil, oregano, basil, and parsley. Stir together until the mixture is combined. It should stick together easily. If it's too sticky, add in more bread crumbs. If it's too dry, add a little more oil or water. Add salt and pepper to taste.

Scoop out 1 tablespoon of the mixture at a time, roll into a ball, and place on the prepared baking sheet. Drizzle with more olive oil for crispier meatballs, then bake for 20 minutes, or until golden brown.

To serve with pasta, cook the pasta according to the package instructions. Warm the marinara sauce in a medium saucepan and right before serving, stir together with the meatballs. Serve with the cooked pasta and Pepita Parmesan, if desired.

To serve as a sandwich, warm the sauce and the meatballs, then toss to just combine. Stuff into a toasted (or untoasted) sub roll and enjoy!

3 PLANT POINTS

Low FODMAP Option:

Limit serving of meatballs to 1½ meatballs if sensitive to GOS. Two chickpea meatballs are considered low FODMAP.

Tomato sauce may contain onion and garlic. If you are sensitive to fructans, look for these low FODMAP tomato sauce options: We like Fody Tomato Basil Pasta Sauce, Fody Marinara Pasta Sauce, and Rao's Homemade Sensitive Marinara Sauce.

Quick Garlic Broccoli

This is less of a recipe and more of a serving suggestion. Steamed broccoli tossed with a little olive oil, minced garlic, salt, pepper . . . and dry mustard. While steaming does lead to the deactivation of myrosinase and therefore stops sulforaphane formation, the addition of dry mustard to cooked broccoli provides a natural source of the enzyme; you get the same benefits of eating it cooked as you would raw.

We recommend using a Microplane grater or garlic press to get the garlic very fine, as you will be enjoying it raw and large pieces of raw garlic can be unpleasant. If you don't own a garlic press or grater, finely mince the garlic with a knife, then use the wide blade to press over the minced garlic, rubbing the blade back and forth to form a paste.

Serves 2
2 cups broccoli florets
1 garlic clove, very finely minced
1 to 2 teaspoons olive oil
¼ teaspoon salt
¼ teaspoon freshly ground black pepper
½ teaspoon dry mustard

Bring a pot of water fitted with a steamer basket to a boil over X heat. Add the broccoli florets and cook for 5 to 7 minutes, until just fork tender, taking care not to overcook.

Remove from the pot and immediately toss with the garlic, olive oil, salt, pepper, and dry mustard. The warmth of the broccoli will gently heat the garlic and oil. Enjoy as is, or at room temperature.

Low FODMAP Option:

Three-quarters cup broccoli florets is low FODMAP. If you're
sensitive to fructose, reduce the total amount of broccoli to 1½ cups.
Omit the garlic and use garlic-infused olive oil (see page 246).

2 PLANT POINTS

Lentil Sloppy Joes

We designed these sandwiches for evenings when you need
something healthy, hearty, and filling.

Serves 2
¼ cup brown or green lentils, rinsed and drained
1 teaspoon olive oil
¼ cup finely chopped onion
½ carrot, finely chopped
½ red bell pepper, finely chopped
¼ cup canned diced tomatoes
2 teaspoons smoked paprika
1 teaspoon garlic powder
1 tablespoon tomato paste
1 teaspoon 100% maple syrup
1 teaspoon Dijon mustard
1 teaspoon apple cider vinegar
¼ teaspoon salt
2 whole-grain buns, for serving
Jicama Fries (page 333), for serving

Add the lentils to a medium saucepan and cover with ¾ cup water.
Bring to a boil over medium-high heat, reduce the heat to low, cover,
and simmer for 25 minutes, or until the lentils are tender.

Heat the olive oil in a large skillet over medium-high heat. Add the onion, carrot, and bell pepper and cook for 5 minutes, or until soft.

Stir in the cooked lentils, tomatoes, paprika, and garlic powder. Cook, stirring occasionally, for another 2 to 3 minutes, until warmed through, then whisk in the tomato paste, maple syrup, Dijon, vinegar, and salt. Simmer for an additional 5 to 10 minutes, until hot and thickened.

Serve on toasted buns with jicama fries.

Low FODMAP Options:

Onion is moderate in fructans. Sub ¼ cup sliced green scallions. Garlic powder is high in fructans. Omit and use 1 teaspoon garlic-infused olive oil (see page 246).

Supercharge It!

Add sauerkraut, pickles, fresh onion, scallions, or avocado to your sandwich.

Make-Ahead Tips:

Cooking the lentils ahead of time will make this recipe come together quickly.

6 PLANT POINTS

Jicama Fries

Jicama is a round root vegetable with a starchy inside that is popular in Mexican cuisine. Tossed with a few classic seasonings, it's our fun twist on baked french fries!

Serves 2

1 small jicama (2½ cups), peeled and sliced into matchsticks

1½ teaspoons olive oil

¼ teaspoon salt

1 teaspoon smoked paprika

½ teaspoon garlic powder

¼ teaspoon freshly ground black pepper

Preheat the oven to 425°F. Line a rimmed baking sheet with foil or parchment paper and set aside.

Place the sliced jicama in a large bowl and add the olive oil. Add in the salt, smoked paprika, garlic powder, and black pepper. Toss until well coated and place in a single layer on the prepared baking sheet.

Bake for 20 minutes, or until slightly crisp. Remove from the oven and serve.

Low FODMAP Options:

A ½-cup serving of fries is low FODMAP.

Omit the garlic powder if sensitive to fructans or garlic.

1 PLANT POINT

Chickpea and Avocado Sandwich

This simple deli-inspired salad sandwich is perfect for busy weekdays. Make at night, then pack separately from sliced sourdough bread to assemble right before eating.

Serves 2

1 cup chickpeas, rinsed and drained

1 large avocado, pitted and roughly chopped

¼ cup chopped cilantro

2 tablespoons finely chopped red onion

1 teaspoon olive oil

Juice of 1 lime

¼ teaspoon salt, plus more to taste

¼ teaspoon freshly ground black pepper, plus more to taste

4 slices sourdough bread, toasted, if desired

Place the chickpeas and avocado in a medium bowl and mash together using a fork or potato masher. Add the cilantro, onion, olive oil, lime juice, salt, and pepper. Season to taste as desired, then serve between toasted sourdough and supercharge toppings of your choice.

Supercharge It!

Add spinach or arugula leaves, microgreens or broccoli sprouts, or sliced tomato.

Low FODMAP Options:

1 cup chickpeas has moderate GOS. Reduce to ½ cup.

1 whole avocado is high in sorbitol. Reduce to ¼ avocado and add 2 tablespoons Dijon mustard.

Red onion is high in fructans. Sub 1 tablespoon scallions or chives.

4 PLANT POINTS

Tuscan Kale Soup

This one-pot soup is thick and oh so satisfying, perfect for weeknights.

Serves 2

1½ tablespoons olive oil or garlic-infused olive oil (see page 246)

½ small white onion, chopped

2 celery ribs, chopped

1 carrot, chopped

½ teaspoon salt, plus more as needed

1 teaspoon dried oregano

½ teaspoon dried basil

½ teaspoon dried thyme

Pinch crushed red pepper flakes, more or less depending on spice preference

One 14.5-ounce can diced tomatoes

2 cups Biome Broth (page 249)

½ cup uncooked quinoa

1 bay leaf

2 large handfuls chopped and cleaned kale

Half of a 14.5-ounce can white beans, such as cannellini beans, great northern beans, or butter beans, drained and rinsed

¼ teaspoon freshly ground black pepper, plus more as needed

Heat the olive oil over medium heat in a medium or large pot or Dutch oven. Add the onion, celery, carrot, and salt. Cook, stirring occasionally, for 3 to 5 minutes, until the onion becomes translucent and the vegetables begin to soften.

Add the oregano, basil, thyme, red pepper flakes, and tomatoes with their juice. Cook, stirring occasionally, for 1 to 2 minutes, until well combined.

Add the broth, 1 cup water, the quinoa and bay leaf. Raise the heat up to medium-high, then bring to a boil. Reduce the heat to low, cover, and simmer for 20 to 25 minutes to allow the flavors to develop.

Uncover, stir in the kale and beans, and cook for about 5 minutes, until the greens are just wilted. Remove bay leaf, season with pepper and more salt, as needed, and serve.

Low FODMAP Option:

Onions are high in fructans. Omit the onion and replace with ½ cup scallions.

White beans are high in GOS. Sub ½ can chickpeas.

Supercharge It!

Top this soup with fresh herbs. We think basil and parsley will taste the best!

Make-Ahead Tips:

Make sure to have your Biome Broth (page 249) prepared ahead of time. For faster meal prep, chop all vegetables ahead of time and store in an airtight container in the fridge.

8 PLANT POINTS

Sunday Pasta

Growing up in an Italian household, Alex always associates Sunday evenings with family and piping-hot bowls of pasta. This Sunday dinner combines a few of our fiber-fueled favorites: tempeh sausage, arugula-lemon pesto, roasted tomatoes, and cashew cream. It takes longer than some of the other recipes to come together, but the extra effort is worth it.

The addition of cashew cream is optional, but it makes for an even more luscious dinner. Cashew cream thickens considerably once cooled, so reheat with a few tablespoons of water to thin.

Serves 4, with leftovers to be enjoyed as desired

Roasted Tomatoes

1 pint cherry tomatoes

1 teaspoon olive oil

Salt and freshly ground black pepper

8 ounces whole-grain spaghetti

Tempeh Sausage

1 tablespoon olive oil

8 ounces tempeh, crumbled

1 teaspoon dried fennel

½ teaspoon dried basil

½ teaspoon dried oregano

¼ teaspoon crushed red pepper flakes

½ teaspoon dried sage

1 garlic clove, minced

1 tablespoon tamari

1 tablespoon 100% maple syrup

1 tablespoon freshly squeezed lemon juice

Arugula-Lemon Pesto

3 cups packed arugula

½ cup walnuts

2 tablespoons nutritional yeast

2 garlic cloves, minced

2 tablespoons freshly squeezed lemon juice

¼ cup vegetable broth or water

⅛ teaspoon salt, plus more if desired

⅛ teaspoon freshly ground black pepper, plus more if desired

1 tablespoon olive oil (optional)

Cashew Cream (page 307; optional), for serving

Make the roasted tomatoes: Preheat the oven to 400°F.

Toss the cherry tomatoes with the olive oil and a pinch of salt and pepper, then place on a rimmed baking sheet. Roast for about 25 minutes, until very reduced and soft. Set aside.

Bring a large pot of salted water to a boil over medium-high heat and add the pasta. Cook until just al dente, reserve 1 cup pasta water, and drain. Set aside.

Make the sausage: Heat the olive oil in a large skillet over medium heat. Add the tempeh and cook for about 5 minutes, stirring often, until the tempeh is browned and crispy.

Add the dried fennel, basil, oregano, red pepper flakes, sage, garlic, tamari, maple syrup and lemon juice. Cook, stirring occasionally, for another 2 to 3 minutes and set aside.

Make the pesto: Place the arugula, walnuts, and nutritional yeast in the base of a food processor and blend until very finely chopped. With the motor running, add in the lemon juice, vegetable broth, salt, and pepper. Drizzle in the olive oil, if desired. Add more salt and pepper to taste.

To assemble, toss the cooked spaghetti with the tomatoes, tempeh sausage, pesto, and cashew cream, if using. Thin with the reserved pasta water, adding 1 tablespoon at a time if needed, until creamy. Serve immediately.

Low FODMAP Options:

5 cherry tomatoes per serving is low in fructans, so if sensitive, then reduce to only 20 cherry tomatoes total, or omit.

Whole-grain spaghetti is high in fructans. Reduce to ½ cup cooked per serving for FODMAP friendly, or use an alternative pasta option, like quinoa.

Garlic is high in fructans. Omit and sub 1 teaspoon garlic-infused olive oil (see page 246) for the sausage and 2 teaspoons for the pesto.

The cashews in the cashew cream are high in GOS and have moderate fructans. Omit the cashew cream if sensitive.

Supercharge It!

Top with Pepita Parmesan (page 301), chopped basil, or chopped parsley.

6 PLANT POINTS

DRINKS, SNACKS, AND DESSERTS

Turmeric Latte

Fresh turmeric is often used in turmeric lattes, but this version uses a dried powder that you likely already have in your pantry. Black pepper might sound weird in a latte, but combining black pepper with the curcumin in turmeric enhances curcumin absorption by up to 2,000 percent, as we discussed in Chapter 4. As the weeks progress, sub in canned coconut milk for a very rich, creamy, and satiating beverage.

Serves 2
2 cups unsweetened almond milk
1 teaspoon vanilla extract
1 tablespoon 100% maple syrup
1 teaspoon ground turmeric
¼ teaspoon ground cinnamon
Pinch ground nutmeg
Pinch ground cardamom
Pinch freshly ground black pepper

In a small pot over medium heat, combine the milk, vanilla, maple syrup, turmeric, cinnamon, nutmeg, cardamom, and pepper. Whisk together and bring to a low boil, then reduce the heat to low and simmer for 5 minutes, stirring occasionally.

Divide into two mugs and serve.

To make an iced latte, place the milk, vanilla, maple syrup, turmeric, cinnamon, nutmeg, cardamom, and pepper in a mason jar with a lid and shake vigorously until well combined. Serve over ice, adding more maple syrup as desired.

Low FODMAP Options:

After Week 2, sub in 1 cup canned coconut milk for the almond milk for a creamier, richer latte.

1 PLANT POINT

White Bean Hummus

All the flavors of Italian pesto in a protein-packed bean dip! Serve with crunchy raw vegetable sticks, seedy crackers, or on toasted sourdough bread.

Makes 4 servings

Half of a 14.5-ounce can white beans (navy, cannellini, great northern), drained and rinsed

½ cup fresh basil

1 garlic clove

2 tablespoons olive oil

1 tablespoon tahini

¼ teaspoon salt

Juice of ½ large lemon

Place the white beans, basil, garlic, olive oil, tahini, salt, and lemon juice in the base of a food processor and process until creamy and smooth.

Low FODMAP Options:

White beans are high in GOS. Sub chickpeas and stick with ¼ cup chickpeas per serving for low FODMAP.

Garlic is high in fructans. Omit and use 1 teaspoon garlic-infused olive oil (see page 246).

Supercharge It!

Add 2 tablespoons hemp seeds to provide a boost of plant protein and healthy fats.

Make-Ahead Tips:

This is a great recipe to make on the weekend for easy snacking throughout the week.

6 PLANT POINTS

Omega-3 Balls

These little balls are packed with plant-based omega-3 fatty acids, hence their name.

Makes 12 balls

½ cup rolled oats

½ cup hemp hearts, plus for more topping, if desired

7 dates, pitted

½ cup walnuts

3 tablespoons almond butter

½ teaspoon vanilla extract

½ teaspoon ground cinnamon

Place the oats, hemp hearts, dates, walnuts, almond butter, vanilla, and cinnamon in the base of a food processor and blend until well combined, scraping down the sides as needed. If the mixture is dry, add 1 tablespoon of water at a time until a dough forms.

Pinch off the dough 1 tablespoon at a time and roll into balls. If the dough is too sticky, add in a little oat flour or place in the fridge to harden.

Continue with the rest of the dough and enjoy as is, or roll into hemp seeds, shredded coconut, and/or very finely chopped walnuts for more texture.

Low FODMAP Options:

Dates have moderate fructans. Reduce the number of dates to 4, so that 1 bite contains ⅓ date. You may need to add 1 to 2 teaspoons maple syrup for sweetness.

Make-Ahead Tips:

Make these ahead of time and store in the fridge for 2 to 3 weeks or in the freezer for up to 4 months. Thaw before enjoying.

5 PLANT POINTS

Strawberry Cheesecake Bites

These bites have been a staple in our house for years. They come together fairly quickly and can be stored in the freezer for whenever you need a quick, yummy dessert. Nuts are nutrition powerhouses and we are using both almonds and cashews to create a luscious, dairy-free cheesecake. Because many of the key ingredients here are high FODMAP, if you are sensitive to GOS or fructans, we suggest making the Coconut Oat Balls (page 250) instead.

Note: If the dates are hard, soak them in warm water for 10 minutes before using, then drain.

Makes 9 bites

Raw Date Crust

1 cup (about 13) pitted dates (red light, f'tan)

1 cup almonds (red light, GOS)

1 tablespoon unsweetened cocoa powder

Pinch salt

Creamy Strawberry Filling

1 cup raw cashews, soaked in warm water for at least 20 minutes, then drained (red light, GOS, f'tan)

1 cup strawberries, chopped
½ cup full-fat canned coconut milk
⅓ cup 100% maple syrup
Juice of 1 large lemon

Make the date crust: Add the dates to the base of a food processor and process until a thick paste forms. Remove and set aside.

Add the almonds, cocoa powder, and salt to the same food processor and process until the nuts are broken down into a fine crumb. Add the date paste back in and process until combined. It should be sticky enough that you can pinch the mixture and it will stick together.

Lightly spray a 12-cup muffin tin with cooking spray, line with muffin liners, or place a thin strip of parchment paper in the bottom of each muffin cup, with enough overhang so the cups can easily be pulled out after being frozen. Place about 1 tablespoon of the crust in the bottom of the muffin tins and press down to fill. Set aside.

Make the filling: Clean out the food processor. Add the cashews, strawberries, coconut milk, maple syrup, and lemon juice to the food processor and puree until very creamy and smooth, scraping down as needed. Depending on your food processor, it may take a few minutes until the cashews are creamy and not gritty.

Evenly pour the filling onto the prepared crust, then place in the freezer for 3 to 4 hours, until hardened. To remove, lightly run a butter knife around the edge of the cheesecakes or pull with the parchment paper overhang.

Because these are no-bake and raw, they don't keep well outside of the freezer. Enjoy leftovers right from the freezer or let thaw for a few minutes before enjoying.

Low FODMAP Option:

Dates are high in fructans. One-third of a date is low FODMAP. If you're sensitive, make the Turmeric Energy Bites (page 310) instead! Almonds are high in GOS. Ten almonds (amount contained in 1 bite) is low FODMAP.

Cashews are high in GOS and fructans. Ten cashews (amount contained in 1 bite) has high GOS and moderate fructans.

5 PLANT POINTS

Snicker Bites

We designed these date bombs to be a quick snack whenever you need something sweet, salty, and satisfying. We call these "snicker bites" because they taste similar to a Snickers bar!

Makes 1 bite
1 date, pitted and halved
1 teaspoon peanut butter
4 to 5 chocolate chips
½ teaspoon sesame seeds

Stuff the date with peanut butter and chocolate chips. Sprinkle with sesame seeds.

Low FODMAP Options:

Dates are high in fructans. If you're sensitive, make the Turmeric Energy Bites (page 310) instead!

3 PLANT POINTS

To view the 5 scientific references cited in this chapter, please visit me online at www.theplantfedgut.com/research/.

Acknowledgments

This has been an incredible, unexpected journey that started with just opening my eyes and my mind to the possibility of things beyond what I was taught in my medical education. Along that path have been numerous people who supported, encouraged, edified, and inspired me.

There are too many of you to mention, but if you've been a part of my life then without a doubt you are one of those people. There are just a few that I'd like to give special mention because, without you, this book would not have been possible.

To my wife, Valarie: I couldn't have done it without you, babe. As in building our home and raising our family, you have once again shown me that together we are so much better than alone. Every time I needed something—whether it was an editor, words of support and encouragement, talking stuff through, time to get stuff done, or sage guidance for a tough choice—you were always there for me. Every single time. I can't tell you how much that means to me, and it makes me love you even more.

To my family, Noreen Johnson, the late Bill Bulsiewicz, Susan and Larry Kobrovsky: You have always been there for me and helped mold me into who I am today. I am eternally grateful for your love and support. I am one fortunate guy to be blessed with such a wonderful family.

To my editor, Lucia Watson: Every single word and action from you from the moment we met has been your belief in this project. You went above and beyond to help me shape my ideas into this book. No matter what happens, I know that we've created something together that's going to help a lot of people.

To my agent, Stephanie Tade: Every day I am grateful for that fateful first meeting and that you decided to take a chance on me. Thank you for believing in this project from the very beginning and being a champion for it all the way through to the finish line. You are simply the best.

To my co-writer, Colleen Martell: I miss our calls, Colleen! Thank you for the having the patience to hear all my crazy ideas and then helping me work through them and shape them over iterations into what this is today. I'm damn proud of our work and can't wait to see what people think.

To my recipe developer, Alexandra Caspero: I feel like you're the secret weapon in this book. There are a lot of books with recipes, but this is some next-level stuff. Thank you for being willing to use my ideas and complex requests to help build the Fiber Fueled 4 Weeks. It's incredible.

To my incredible Plant Fed Gut team, Michelle and Ali at Soul Camp; Jonathan and everyone at Digital Natives; Lalita Ballesteros, my course developer; Sarah Eustis, my intern: I'd write an entire page to each of you if I could. I think you guys know how I feel . . . I have the best team supporting me and this project. I am continuously blown away by how you've each gone above and beyond for me. I appreciate you so much.

To my publicity and marketing team, Anne and Farin at Avery; Rena and Natalie at Stanton: Thank you for your tireless efforts. I am sincerely grateful for everything you've done to help me spread this message that I so passionately believe in.

Megan Newman and Suzy Swartz at Avery: Thank you for your belief in and commitment to this project.

Simon Hill from *The Plant Proof Podcast*: Thanks for giving me a shot and always being so supportive. The decision to write this book really came from meeting you, my friend.

Robby and Cyrus from *Mastering Diabetes*: You're just the best and constantly went above and beyond for me. Thank you.

Drs. Nick Shaheen, John Pandolfino, Balfour Sartor, Doug Drossman, and Peter Kahrilas: Thank you for investing your time into my mentorship. I admire every one of you. You have shaped me as a physician, as a scientist, and as a man.

To all my friends on social media: I wish I could call every single one of you out by name. You know who you are! I am so grateful for our friendship and your support of this book and my platform. It's crazy to get to work alongside my own personal health heroes. Thank you for inspiring me.

Last, but certainly not least . . .

To my children: Daddy loves you! And I will always love you! You are my greatest gift and my most proud accomplishment.

INDEX